AGING WITH CARE

AGING WITH CARE

Your Guide to Hiring and Managing Caregivers at Home

Amanda Lambert and Leslie Eckford

ROWMAN & LITTLEFIELD
Lanham • Boulder • New York • London

The information provided in this book is designed to provide helpful information on the subjects discussed. References are provided for informational purposes only and do not constitute endorsement of any websites, companies, products, organizations or programs. Readers should be aware that the websites listed in this book may change.

Published by Rowman & Littlefield
A wholly owned subsidiary of The Rowman & Littlefield Publishing Group, Inc.
4501 Forbes Boulevard, Suite 200, Lanham, Maryland 20706
www.rowman.com

6 Tinworth Street, London, SE11 5AL, UK

British Library Cataloguing in Publication Information Available

Library of Congress Cataloging-in-Publication Data

Names: Lambert, Amanda, author. | Eckford, Leslie, author.
Title: Aging with care : your guide to hiring and managing caregivers at home / Amanda Lambert and Leslie Eckford.
Description: Lanham : Rowman & Littlefield, [2017] | Includes bibliographical references and index.
Identifiers: LCCN 2017013069 (print) | LCCN 2017031876 (ebook) | ISBN 9781442281646 (electronic) | ISBN 9781442281639 (cloth : alk. paper) | ISBN 9781538125991 (pbk : alk. paper)
Subjects: LCSH: Home care services—Evaluation. | Caregivers. | Older people—Care. | Home nursing.
Classification: LCC RA645.3 (ebook) | LCC RA645.3 .L36 2017 (print) | DDC 362.2/4—dc23
LC record available at https://lccn.loc.gov/2017013069

∞ ™ The paper used in this publication meets the minimum requirements of American National Standard for Information Sciences Permanence of Paper for Printed Library Materials, ANSI/NISO Z39.48-1992.

Printed in the United States of America

To our parents and our families.
And to the countless caregivers who provide
compassionate and dedicated care to elders.

CONTENTS

PREFACE

Throughout *Aging with Care* are stories about real people who are dealing with issues of aging at home and managing life with the help of professional caregivers. While these are all real stories, all identifying information such as names and locations has been changed to protect privacy. Some stories are based on composites of real people whom we have known or worked with over the years. Other stories are told by the actual people from our interviews for the purpose of this book. We are deeply grateful for their willingness to share their thoughts and feelings. Their experiences have deepened our appreciation of this challenging journey. We hope our readers will feel the same.

ACKNOWLEDGMENTS

This book came into being from its earliest stages to its finishing touches with the good guidance of our first reader and "editor extraordinaire," Lisa Goldstein Kieda. We thank Lisa for her constant interest, positive energy, incomparable humor, and, above all, friendship. We also extend our appreciation to our agent, Gina Panettieri, who believed in the importance and relevance of our book.

INTRODUCTION

Waking Up to a Nightmare: Leslie's Story

"Hello, Marsha?"

"Yes, hello, Leslie, how are you?"

"I'm fine, thank you. First, I want to tell you how grateful I am to you for staying while my mother was sick the last two days and nights. I know that wasn't easy, and, well, me and my family, we all really appreciate you doing that, and how hard that is on you to be away from your own family during that time, and really how much you have done for my dear parents."

"Well, sure, you know, I love your parents, and it was no trouble, really."

"And, now, Marsha, I need you to pay attention very carefully. You are fired as of today, this minute."

(Pause)

"Is there a warrant out for me?"

This was one of the most difficult conversations that I have had in recent memory. I fired a caregiver who had become like a member of the family, whom I had entrusted with the care of my dear, funny, difficult, beloved old parents. I fired this person, a lovely older woman with a sweet smile, kind blue eyes, and bleached blonde hair, a person who had come highly recommended by a trusted healthcare provider and friends of my parents, who had given my mother and father good care, often going above and beyond my expectations. This caregiver had been providing 'round the clock, twenty-four-hour care to my elderly parents who live in their own home and have mobility needs and memory problems.

Why did I fire her? Credit card fraud and stealing checks, jewelry, medications, and food (not a meal or two, but whole weeks' worth of groceries). And as time went on, there was neglect of my parents' care: lack of hygiene, not giving essential medications for weeks at a time. There's more, but I won't go into that now. You get the idea. It was a worst-case scenario for the people for whom I hold the greatest loyalty and love. And I'm the one who set it up and arranged to pay for it with their money.

The problem is that I thought I could do this job of monitoring my parents' care very well. After all, I am an RN and a Licensed Clinical Social Worker and have specialized in geriatric mental health for many years. But I was wrong. I live over two thousand miles away from my parents. I visit my parents three to four times a year in addition to making video calls and phone calls. However, that was not enough. After the required period of wallowing in guilt and anger and wanting to give up, I was bound and determined that I would learn how to make it work.

This story happened over two years ago. My parents still live at home; they still have 'round the clock caregivers. However, almost everything about their arrangement is different now. I no longer hand over the reins to anyone for any part of their care without very thorough scrutiny. I have completely changed how I manage their living and care situation. I have changed it from the ground up and with the blinders off. It has certainly not been easy, but their care and my attitude about managing it have undergone a major evolution.

After we had been taken to the cleaners by the unscrupulous caregiver, I had briefly mentioned some of my caregiving catastrophe to my friend and colleague, Amanda Lambert. As any good friend would do, she was kind and sympathetic, and as we were both busy people, we agreed to talk more at a later time. I knew that she was a geriatric care manager, but because I also had much geriatric experience, I hadn't thought previously of asking her advice about my parents' care. One thing I knew we had in common from our professional work together was that we are both passionate and dedicated to supporting people's need to age in the community, in their own home and familiar surroundings whenever possible.

In an e-mail, Amanda said casually, "Hey, do you want to write a book about caregivers?" Thus began a conversation that revealed a great disconnect between us about our approach to hiring caregivers. Amanda explained to me that she would have never recommended that I hire caregivers privately. And I, even after this terrible experience, still prefer to hire someone myself rather than through a private care agency. We realized that our great debate is also one that many other people are having. Every day, more and more families are facing the questions: "How can I manage to work/raise my family/commute to another city and take care of mom or dad?," "Who can we hire to help mom or dad with their daily needs?," and "How in the world are we going to pay for it?" Because, in case you haven't heard, the geriatric tsunami is heading here fast.

I

TWO APPROACHES TO HIRING CAREGIVERS

Amanda and Leslie have always agreed that if there is a safe and work-able way for an elder to stay and live at home, it is the best option for a number of reasons. Familiar surroundings offer a level of comfort and emotional security that cannot be easily replaced in an assisted living or nursing home setting. We will share more about the consequences for the elderly of moving from home further along in this chapter.

We are staunch advocates of the concept and practice of "aging in place." Aging in place means living at home as one ages, rather than moving to a residential environment, such as assisted living or a nursing home. Our stance is not based solely on our opinion. In survey after survey by AARP over multiple years, the majority of older American adults indicate that they adamantly want to stay in their present homes.[1] However, choosing to stay in one's home with assistive care is usually a challenge to put into practice and may not be the perfect solution for everyone. Is it the right decision for you or your family member?

Many families, feeling that they are unprepared, have gone headlong into the process of hiring caregivers. They may be pressured by medical circumstances or crisis. A daughter may make a sudden discovery about how poorly an elder family member is doing at home. Others may be acting on the observations and well-meaning advice from friends, neigh-bors, or landlords who report signals of decline. Making major life-changing decisions with a clock ticking ("We've got to decide where dad is going before he is discharged from the hospital this weekend!") can increase the risk of making choices that you may later regret. We shared Leslie's cautionary tale in the introduction and her perspective of being a family member who has had a wild hired caregiving adventure. Now we will hear about Amanda's professional journey and how she came to take a significant role in choosing to hire caregivers for her clients.

AMANDA'S STORY

I love working with elders. From the moment I managed a small Elderhostel program in New Hampshire, I was hooked. I am fascinated by topics on healthy aging, aging in place, and housing and support services for low-income elders. I also love stories of amazing athletic feats by older adults! Many years later the landscape has changed and is evolving at a mind-blowing rate. Caregiving is one of the most important issues of aging in the twenty-first century.

I am a nationally Certified Care Manager and Master Guardian and a professional member of the Aging Life Care Association. I have worked for over twenty-five years with elders in a variety of settings, most recently as president and owner of my own care management company in Salt Lake City, Utah. I monitor and manage the care of several elders and work with numerous home health and home care agencies and the many dedicated and passionate people who choose this work.

What is a geriatric care manager? I am a surrogate decision maker, de facto family member, and manager all rolled into one. I have clients with dementia, Parkinson's disease, multiple sclerosis, chronic medical conditions, and mental health disorders, just to name a few. Ultimately my job is to make sure that my clients are well cared for and safe, and let's not forget the often overlooked importance of quality of life. Keeping someone safe is one of the first reasons families hire caregivers, but what about these questions: How does my client feel about having a caregiver come into his or her home? What is important to this person? Can the elder even verbalize what they want or need?

As I begin the process of finding a caregiver for a client, unlike Leslie, I will not look at hiring outside a licensed and bonded agency. I work for an independent geriatric care management company that has no ties to other healthcare companies or agencies. I am at liberty to pick the agencies that I feel will do the best job for my client, and if they don't and something goes wrong, I can hold the agency accountable and they will have the responsibility of handling it. There are companies that are designed to help you find private caregivers, but that is not the same as a caregiving agency. For example, Care.com is a successful online company that assists with finding privately hired caregivers (or connecting you to an array of local caregiving agencies) and also provides options to pay for background checks and an online format for paying taxes.

Deciding to use a home care agency also comes with potential problems. I am well aware of the high turnover rate of caregivers and the difficulty of finding the right person for the job who can accommodate a client's schedule and personal preferences. It is against federal law to discriminate in hiring a caregiver or anyone else based on a protected category such as race, national origin, or sex, but this does not prevent some people from making such requests. So in other words, my role is to pick the person who will be the best match for my client considering my client's personality, needs, wants, personal preferences in terms of temperament, quality of life, and safety. And then it is my responsibility to make sure that this person remains a good fit even though my client may not be able to verbalize problems or concerns. Sound impossible? Add to these challenges the cost of providing care or limits on minimum hours an agency will provide care. Find a good caregiver that is the perfect fit? Chances are they will leave for better pay or to continue their education and then you are back to the search again.

THE AGING TSUNAMI

The United States and the rest of the world are facing an aging superstorm. The implications are so profound and so significant that we are just beginning to awaken from our slumber to realize we have a problem. In fact, we have many problems associated with an aging population that is living longer despite chronic medical conditions, Alzheimer's disease, and other age-related conditions.

The older population—persons sixty-five years or older—numbered 39.6 million in 2009 (the latest year for which data are available). They represented 12.9 percent of the U.S. population, about one in every eight Americans. By 2030, there will be about 72.1 million older persons, more than twice the number in 2000. People aged sixty-five and older represented 12.4 percent of the population in the year 2000 and are expected to grow to be 19 percent of the population by 2030.[2]

Families are in a panic and the aging industry is struggling to fill the need for caregivers of our aging population. Paid caregivers are rallying for improved benefits, overtime pay, and increased wages. Whether these costs will be passed on to the consumer remains to be seen. Today about two million home care aides assist eleven million elders and people with disabilities.[3] These aides fall into two formal occupations tracked by the U.S. Department of Labor: home health aides and home care aides. Both occupations are expected to grow by nearly 50 percent over the decade from 2012 to 2022, a rate nearly five times higher than the rate of overall job growth in the economy.[4]

So why are we so passionate about elders staying at home? Well, have you been to a nursing home lately? The average assisted living facility? We have been to lots of them. Yes, there are some fine ones, but the best ones are usually few and far between, have long waiting lists, and can be very expensive. And besides, 80 to 90 percent of elders state they would like to remain in their homes for as long as possible.[5] Ten years or so ago, we greatly admired the lovely three levels of care facilities (referred to as "three tiered" care or continuing retirement communities by the industry). They offer independent living apartments as well as assisted living apartments for you to grow into, and then, if you need it, you can stay in their top of the line skilled nursing unit right on the premises. Nowadays, however, they have more stringent entry requirements, and you can forget about having your application accepted by them if you do not look like a walking active senior advertisement.

Depending on the location and the market, you may find getting into an assisted living or three-tiered option is easier or harder to get into than elsewhere. In some areas, it can be more difficult to find assisted living facilities to take you if you are already in a wheelchair. A daughter-in-law confided to us that she rushed her in-laws into moving in to a retirement community that they liked because it had the reputation, as she put it, as a "walk in, roll out": the admissions requirements were such that if you couldn't walk in on your own steam, you would not be admitted. Once you were in, you could stay there until they had to roll you out. On the other hand, a nurse in another region of the country told us that at the assisted living unit where she works, the residents living there currently have changed dramatically in the level of care that they need; they are more like the residents of a skilled nursing home ten years ago with advanced medical and mobility problems. It differs greatly by location and by the zoning laws that govern the area in which the facility is built. One person we know had toured a really nice, very pricey three-tiered retirement community for her parents in their late seventies. It had all the bells and whistles, such as a full program of activities, lectures, day trips, and concierge services. She loved it and thought her parents would too. She mentioned to the director that though her father continued to be spry, her mother had had a stroke and was in a wheelchair, requiring some assistance with home care from a caregiver. She was told that her parents would not be able to move into that independent level together. The same facility allows couples who are active to move into the independent level and if one starts to need care, they are both allowed to stay in that level with added care (usually hired by the family and with added expense). But they cannot have any limitations at the outset. The director suggested to this couple that they would have to live in separate apartments (independent or assisted living) because their apartments were not designed for two residents, or the mother could live in the nursing home unit. These rules may be understandable from a zoning and legal perspective, but it can be confusing and frustrating for people and their families to take in when making such an important and life-changing decision.

In fact, "the third tier," the skilled nursing option of the three-tier retirement community, appears to be fading out of existence and is no longer part of the design in some newer senior communities. A senior who lives in such a retirement community told us that many seniors themselves don't want to move into a place where there are "a lot of old people." "We want to be around healthy people, like us." Sadly, the older generation does not want visible reminders of what may lay ahead as well. For many considering the move, the "active senior lifestyle" communities exemplified by Del Webb's Sun City are highly appealing. These beautifully maintained senior residences are very tempting with all the amenities: golf, exercise studios, pickle ball courts, shuffleboard, and more. But as healthy older adults advance in age, they too may start to require assistance, necessitating another move, one that might be more difficult to make. We have met many formerly "healthy lifestyle" individuals (skiers, runners, hikers, teetotalers, nonsmokers, and the like) who, beyond their control, have developed chronic, debilitating disease in their old age. None of us has a crystal ball. If choosing and investing in the expensive active senior lifestyle residence as a home for the end of life, one must plan emotionally and financially for the realistic possibility that it might not be one's last home.

When you get down to the brass tacks, the transition from living at home to moving to a facility at an advanced age can result in some negative and heartbreaking consequences. It is widely known in the geriatric research literature that rates of depression among those who have moved to a nursing home are very high, hovering around 30 percent of long-term care residents.[6] It's not uncommon for people to start to fail, medically and emotionally, after this move. We have met very few older adults who have said to us, "Hey, I'm super excited! I'm finally moving to the assisted living! I finally get to go to the nursing home!" No, it doesn't usually go like that. It's more like someone is being brave, bracing themselves for the spoonful of castor oil or worse, the firing squad. When Leslie had finished graduate school, she went for a job interview at a very well-respected assisted living facility. While waiting in the lobby for her interview, a resident walked through the ornately decorated but largely empty space. Leslie recognized this woman as a former patient from her work on a geriatric psychiatry unit. The resident also recognized Leslie and smiled. This intelligent elder lady looked transformed from the time of her hospital stay: she was well dressed and coiffed, moving with greater ease. She looked Leslie in the eye and with a sweet smile said, "It's nice and quiet in here isn't it?" Leslie smiled back and said, "Yes it is." The resident, with some well-practiced sarcasm, responded as she turned and left the lobby, "Yes, nice and quiet . . . just like a morgue."

Of course, we have been there to support the elders who do make this move and help them find features in their new home that resonate for them in a good way. We've seen that a positive outcome is more likely when the elder themself makes the decision to move from their home to another living arrangement, rather than being pressured to do so from a hospital bed. As advocates for the elderly and their children, we support families to protect elders from the risks associated with continued physical and mental decline. Occasionally the only viable solution is to choose to move from an unmanageable home environment. We can assist the elder in the transition by monitoring for and getting help to treat depression. We search with them for the human factor that will make the difference. We may advocate for living at home, but we are realists too. We know that in some situations, it is simply not possible to avoid the change.

But what is it really like to make the choice to stay at home and need the help of home care providers? Is it really so much better? Picture the perfect transition as you age: you are a person who has always been independent, managing your life and your work with enthusiasm and energy. You have found yourself with the blessing of good friends and relationships, perhaps have raised a family, been a reliable and valued member of the community, and an employee and/or employer. You have enjoyed relatively good health and been active in sports and exercise.

Then, as you age, you good naturedly recognize the normal slowing down, accept the deaths and illnesses of your close friends philosophically, and mature with grace and wisdom as you consider your own end. As your physical and mental slowing increases, you consider the thoughtful suggestions of your adult children and friends that a little help is in order and agree to look at all the options. You agree that a caregiver is needed and you and your family seek and find a wonderful person who will fill that role.

What is the real role of the paid caregiver and what have you gotten yourself into? Here are some of your thoughts: I'm a grown person and this is my house. Why do they have to be here all the time? They sit around a lot, and I'm paying for this? Why are they moving my furniture around? I like it and want it just the way it was. How can I find things if my kitchen has been rearranged? I don't need this, and I sure don't want this. I can go to the store by myself. What if someone I know sees me with this person? They will think I am old. Since when do I need someone to go into the bathroom with me and wipe me? Why do they have to be in the shower with me? I can do it myself! Can't a person have a little privacy? The reality of having a paid caregiver in your or your family member's home can be a startling change. Clearly, even if someone is choosing to stay at home and has the house and finances to make it work, it is a big decision and still a complicated transition in life.

At this point, a professional perspective can be greatly valuable. As previously mentioned, we are two geriatric professionals who do not necessarily agree on the best approach. However, we are certain that our different points of view can be helpful to those embarking on this path.

CONSIDER YOUR DECISION ON A CONTINUUM

So here you have two colleagues who approach how to hire a caregiver in two different ways. We want to make sure that you know that there is not one right way to do this. So much depends on the details of your individual situation. You may combine both options in your care plan for your loved one. It may be helpful to consider all the pros and cons on a continuum. The inevitability of change may necessitate a transition from an agency to hiring privately or from hiring privately to an agency or a combination of both. It is important to recognize, however, that dramatic changes in health or finances can also indicate that the home option is no longer viable and it may be time to move.

The bottom line for Leslie:

- Hiring from an agency is more expensive. You do have to factor in paying wages and taxes, your elder's home insurance may need an upgrade, and of course all the expenses related to the upkeep and maintenance of your parent's home. But you have more freedom to negotiate what the wage is for an individual caregiver based on their experience and training. That can be a win-win for both employer and caregiver as they generally receive very low wages from an agency.
- You get to decide who is going to be the caregiver, not who is available at the agency that day. This not only gives you and your parent more control over the hiring decision, it can add to peace of mind. This can be a very important and empowering step in the transition from being independent to accepting that you are dependent in some ways on another person.
- There is less turnover. People who work for families privately tend to be happier with the consistency and stability of the job, are usually better paid than when they work at an agency, and have the opportunity to develop loyalty to their client. We started with an agency before my parents needed twenty-four-hour care. But when my parents would finally connect with an individual caregiver, she would be transferred to another case or only worked occasional shifts. Invariably, they did not like the replacement caregiver(s). Some weeks there would be three or more different people coming to help my parents. This added stress and conflict to an already not

Table 1.1.   Leslie's Perspective: The Pros and Cons of Hiring Privately

Pros	Cons
Hiring from an agency is more expensive, especially if you need less than twenty-four-hour care.	There are hidden costs in home insurance, payroll taxes, and unemployment if you fire someone.
You decide who the caregiver will be.	Hiring, firing, and managing caregivers is *very* time consuming and stressful.
There is less turnover and more loyalty.	You, your parent, and your siblings may disagree strongly about who is the right caregiver.
A consistent caregiver means that the care and communication are better.	Consistency is great, but you may find you have hired the "okay, but not quite right" caregiver and keep that person in the job because it is too much of a hassle to find a replacement.
An array of online services and brick and mortar businesses offer a small employer ways to check backgrounds and do pre-employment drug screenings to protect families.	These essential activities to hiring still take time and effort for family members to conduct.
You and your family member develop a relationship and a rapport with the caregiver that you hire yourselves. You may have the same caregiver(s) for years at a time, which promotes the sense of family that many people have with the best caregivers.	You and your family member also develop loyalties and feelings for the caregiver, which makes it harder to respond impartially to situations that arise in which you need to question the caregiver's actions or intentions. If you become close and work well with an agency caregiver, you will have to pay a very large "finder's fee" to hire them away from the agency.
You and your family have more control over what is going on day in and day out. If you are more of a DIYer or like to be very hands-on in your involvement with your aging parent, this the option for you.	If you have no experience in managing the work of other people, scheduling, or conflict management, you will be better off getting the support of an agency. You are responsible for any mistakes that happen on your watch.
When someone calls in sick, you may have one or more caregivers who like to have extra shifts and cover. If you don't have backups in your system, you can call an agency.	If your family member is not on the regular schedule for an agency, it can be difficult to get coverage on short notice.
You can contract out the payroll. A payroll company or online service can provide simple online time clock systems that increase honest and accurate time keeping. They will take care of holiday hours, taxes, cutting checks, or making direct deposits.	It can be expensive, but shopping around will help you find a good deal. Remember that some banks have online payroll systems for small businesses, and there are many independent online options. With a small operation, this can be one of the best decisions that you make.

If you have a very close relationship with
your parent or need to know every aspect
of their care immediately, you may feel
more comfortable with hiring privately.

If there has been strain or pain in your
relationship with your parent before they
needed more help, you may want more outside
support, such as hiring a geriatric care manager,
to manage their care.

ideal situation. We heard a story of a daughter who had hired
through an agency and was feeling happy when her mother told her
that she really liked a particular agency caregiver. But she later
discovered that the caregiver was not interested or able to get her
mother to do some basic bathing or showering. She was more interested in getting along with the mother than making sure that she got
dressed every day.

• Consistent caregivers mean that the care and the communication are
better. Ever play that telephone game in which one person whispers
a story in the ear of the person next to them and then that person
whispers it to the one next to them, and it goes on and on to other
people around the circle? The last person tells what they heard and
it is hysterically funny because it is so completely changed from the
original story. But it is not funny at all when your communication
about your parent's care becomes confused or, what seems to happen more frequently, the message simply doesn't make it to the
caregiver at all. Communication about the needs of an elder person
requiring care, especially if you live a distance away or have a job
that makes it difficult for you to call at certain hours, is challenging
under the best circumstances. Add to that a chain of command, such
as needing to go through the shift supervisor of the care agency who
will then relay the message to the caregiver or trying to discuss a
complicated situation directly to a caregiver that you don't know. I
have encountered the "it's not my job" mentality on occasion with
agency caregivers who know they won't be there for more than a
shift or two, so why should they care if my mother doesn't have
something done the way that will make her feel more secure? Medication changes can take days to occur, doctor's appointments can be
missed, or worse. My parents' caregivers know my parents and
what is "normal" for them and what isn't. They know when to call
me if something isn't right. They know the history in a more meaningful way than the caregiver who is covering for just a day or two.

The bottom line for Amanda:

- There is a reality about selecting caregivers that people don't like to talk about. The fact is that many people have preferences . . . and prejudices. I have had clients who flat out state what characteristics they want or don't want in a caregiver that may have nothing to do with compatibility or personality, or they have trouble hearing and request a caregiver whose native language is English. I had one client tell me: "Don't send anyone who is fat!" Clients tell me they want someone who is liberal or they want someone who is conservative. Do you really want the task of weeding out perfectly good caregivers just because of a seemingly superficial and immutable characteristic? An agency cannot, as mentioned previously, discriminate or hire based on federally protected categories, further complicating the likelihood of compatibility. My role is to pick the person who will be the best match for my client considering their

Table 1.2.   Amanda's Perspective: The Pros and Cons of Hiring a Professional Care Agency

Pros	Cons
Selecting the caregiver is the agency's responsibility.	There can be trial and error to find the right person, which can be disruptive and intrusive. There is more staff turnover at agencies.
Last-minute scheduling changes (and they *will* happen with an agency or without) are handled by the agency.	You never know who you will get.
All payroll taxes, insurance, holiday pay, and mileage are paid by the agency.	These costs are passed on to the consumer in the form of higher hourly rates.
The agency is responsible for liability insurance to protect against lawsuits, theft, neglect, and injuries.	There are limits to that liability. But there are limits to liability with private insurance as well.
Your time is precious. Do you really have the time to conduct a small business? Because that is what managing outside caregivers takes in an ongoing way. Let an agency handle it.	You may not like the way an agency deals with their employees or you for that matter. The little details that can sometimes go unattended can be very frustrating. You could show them how to better run their business!
When you notice something wrong, the care isn't what you expect, or the elder doesn't like the caregiver, you go the agency to make a complaint or request a change.	Expect that changes can sometimes be slow if staffing is tight.

personality, needs, wants, and personal preferences as long as those preferences do not run afoul of federal law.

- The call comes in the middle of the night or while you are at work, out to dinner with friends, at the movies, or on vacation: a caregiver is unable to make their shift. A good, reputable agency will fill that shift even if the administrator must to do it themselves. The agency is absolutely responsible for filling that shift and hopefully you can go back to sleep knowing that your family member will have some-one to be there. At least in some cases you may have the option of filling that shift yourself or with another family member if you don't want a strange caregiver coming to the home.

- This should be subtitled: "What a Headache!" Payroll taxes, insu-rance, liability insurance, holiday pay, mileage, background checks, and on and on. If this is your idea of a hobby then go for it, other-wise leave these details to an agency. A reputable home care agency in Salt Lake City told me that in fifteen years of business they have had one lawsuit from a caregiver that was dismissed and never went to court and a total of three thefts, all of which were resolved and the clients reimbursed. However, even with an agency, abuse, theft, fraud, and neglect do happen and indications are that it is vastly underreported. According to the AARP Bulletin,[7] only fifteen states require agencies to conduct periodic in-home reviews to make sure aides are doing their job. There are no federal regulations covering home care workers other than standards for care provided under Medicaid.

- Coping with an aging family member is stressful and time consum-ing. Most people don't have the time to add the additional respon-sibility of managing the small business of caregiving. There is no question that time will be spent monitoring the agency and the caregivers themselves, but it will be much less time. If the agency doesn't meet your requirements, fire them and start with another one. Meet the administrator and care managers of the agency. We will talk more in a later chapter about how to find the best agency. Having a good relationship with the staff of an agency where com-munication is open and honest is priceless.

- Mistakes will happen. This statement should be in bold type and placed on your refrigerator. When things go wrong, the most impor-tant thing is having an agency that will take full responsibility for those errors without rancor, defensiveness, or disagreement. They will make it right. If mistakes happen on your watch with the caregivers you have hired, who is responsible? Much of that responsibility will be yours and you must be prepared to accept that burden and deal with it to the best of your ability.

FINDING THE WAY HOME

As you can see, we have really different thoughts about how to go about hiring a caregiver. We understand that families have to find their own path to a home care solution that ultimately meets the goals of everyone involved, not anyone else's. There truly is more than one way home. This process is unique to each family. It can be an opportunity for much creative problem solving or it can be a devastating decline to the end. There is no judgment if you start with one approach and move to another. Or you may have a final realization that the best choice is to make the move to a well-researched care community. As the oldest daughter of elderly parents who are beginning to need extra care recently said to us, "No one told me to expect this part of life. It is so complicated for me and my brothers and my parents. But I guess that is what life brings to us all, learning something new."

TAKEAWAY POINTS FOR THIS CHAPTER

- Anticipate and expect that if you don't need in-home care now, you will in the future. Start a family discussion so that when the time comes you won't be scrambling during a crisis.
- Identify and investigate home care agencies and online caregiver services so you have an idea of who you feel comfortable hiring.
- Home care agency pros:

  - The agency finds the caregiver. When mistakes happen, a good agency will make it right.
  - Replacement caregivers are identified and scheduled in case of missed visits.

- Liability and background checks are provided. Payroll and taxes are handled by the agency.
- Your time is precious. Do you really want to spend the time and incur the stress of hiring and firing?

- Home care agency cons:

  - Lots of staff turnover. Find a good caregiver and they may leave.
  - There are limits to liability insurance.
  - Background checks are not airtight. Costs for liability insurance, background checks, and payroll are passed on to the consumer.
  - You may not like who the agency picks or how employees are treated.

- Hiring caregivers privately pros:

  - Less expensive to the consumer.
  - More control over who is hired.
  - Potentially better rapport because you are managing, which could translate to less turnover and more loyalty.
  - You can contract out payroll, background checks, and other pre-employment screenings.

- Hiring caregivers privately cons:

  - There are hidden costs of insurance, payroll, and unemployment if you fire someone.
  - Time and stress of managing, hiring, and firing.
  - Disagreements in the family about who to hire.
  - These efforts take time and contracting out payroll can be expensive. It is more difficult to handle problems impartially because you are the one dealing with issues.

- There is no one right way. Evaluate your situation and take the time to make an informed decision. Be flexible and change course if need be.

2

GETTING STARTED

How Much Home Care Do You Need?

Knowing if or when to begin considering care in the home can be complicated. Typically, an event or trigger can be the precipitating factor for family members or even the elder themselves to realize that help is needed. In this chapter, we talk about some of the typical triggers that may occur and provide a Home Care Needs Scale to identify more specifically what tasks may be required. We will start with what may initially appear as small changes that can reveal bigger problems.

Before we get to the Home Care Needs Scale, we will help you conquer some of the jargon that comes along with this journey before it trips you up. The term "home care" needs to be distinguished from "home health care." It's not uncommon for people to get these concepts mixed up. When someone is told by the doctor or nurse that "a nurse will come by the house" to check on their family member, their first response might be to be very happy that the doctor has this whole home care thing figured out. They might be tempted to think that the medical order for home health care will be a longer-term solution. It won't be. The term "home health care" designates services ordered by a medical doctor that are usually paid for by health insurance (such as Medicare) and include medical interventions such as nursing, physical and occupational therapy, and speech therapy that are scheduled as brief visits (such as for one hour) and that are time limited (such as for sixty days to resolve a specific condition, like the healing of a surgical wound, or continued home physical therapy after a hip replacement).[1] It is advisable early in the process to check on Medicare coverage and see what short-term services may be available in the home.

"Home care," in contrast, also known as private duty or personal care, can be an ongoing service. Home care is not covered by health insurance and is an out-of-pocket expense, although it can be covered by a long-term care insurance policy if one has privately purchased such a policy. If you have one, make sure you check the specifics of your long-term care insurance policy because many require a ninety-day waiting period. Some other commonly used terms for describing these private home care services are nonmedical care, personal care, private duty, custodial care, or companionship care. Under the term "home care," paid individuals doing the care may have a Certified Nursing Assistant (CNA) license, but this is typically not required. Tasks that can be provided include the following: companionship, cooking, cleaning, transportation, medication, leisure activities, and assistance with bathing and grooming. Please see table 2.1 describing the difference between Medicare and Medicaid coverage.

We have devised the Home Care Needs Scale to assist you in assessing what care can be done by a family or friend versus a professional caregiver; what activities, such as medication management or bathing, are most important to the particular individual and the family; and in what areas there can be flexibility, such as scheduling and allowing that there be rotating caregivers rather than relying on only one individual. We share many stories of elders who need home care because while every situation is different, some of these people and experiences that we have known may resonate with you and your family's situation. The Home Care Needs Scale will help you determine if staying at home is a realistic option while bringing into sharper focus the specific tasks that may not only increase safety, but also quality of life.

HOME CARE NEEDS SCALE

Keep in mind that levels of care can fluctuate. Your father may be returning home from a couple of weeks in rehab after knee surgery and will likely continue to progress even more when he returns to his familiar home surroundings. If he was managing well at home before the surgery,

Table 2.1. Medicare and Medicaid: Who Pays for What?

Medicare	Medicaid
Medicare is a federally funded insurance program for people over the age of sixty-five. Income and assets are irrelevant.	Medicaid is a federally and state-funded health insurance program for people of all ages with low income and few assets. Medicaid coverage varies from state to state.
For older people, Medicare can be very helpful in providing temporary services in the home when certain conditions are met. These services are time limited, but can in some cases prevent the need for skilled nursing, longer hospitalization, or residential rehabilitation. Usually, a home health care agency coordinates the services your doctor orders for you.	Some Medicaid programs pay for your care directly in the home. Others use private insurance companies to provide Medicaid coverage.
All people with Medicare Part A and/or Part B who meet all of these conditions are covered for limited-time home health services: • You must be under the care of a doctor and you must be getting services under a plan of care established and reviewed regularly by a doctor. • A doctor must certify one or more of these: 　• Intermittent skilled nursing care (other than just drawing blood) 　• Physical therapy, speech-language pathology, respiratory therapy, or continued • The home health agency caring for you must be Medicare certified. • A doctor must certify that you're homebound. The definition of homebound is that you would not be able to leave the house without significant assistance. You may leave home for medical treatment or short, infrequent absences for nonmedical reasons, like attending religious services. You can still get home health care if you attend adult day care.	Unlike Medicare coverage of home health care or regular Medicaid long-term care nursing home coverage, Medicaid waiver programs aren't limited to medical care and their coverage doesn't run out when a person's medical condition stabilizes. The purpose of these waiver programs is to keep people out of nursing homes for as long as possible because nursing home care is more expensive than providing support in a home-based setting.

his needs for home care are probably temporary. In a contrasting scenario, a seventy-three-year-old woman who is also recovering from surgery and rehab may have gotten the attention of the health care team and her family while in the hospital because of her difficulty with managing simple tasks, such as needing help dressing or opening food tray items. The hospital stay is often a time when the older adult or family member may realize how difficult it has been for a person to remember to take pills on time, that they are not bathing and dressing the way they normally would, or how socially isolated they have become.

Another important point: a person's ability to manage is not always linear or straightforward. Don't assume that you can check all the boxes in one section and then your family's situation stays only at that level. Aging and disability can be fluid or sudden, static for long periods or short periods, and unique to the individual involved. If, for example, you can check the first three categories for level one, but there was that one time that your parent decided to go out in the backyard to check on the sprinkler system at 4 a.m. and the neighbor called you, you need to consider level two for safety reasons.

Level One: Simple, Limited Time Home Care

Triggers for level one:

- Moira's mother Jeanine has always been a fabulous cook. While growing up, friends would come over, and they all loved to stay for her mother's delicious, comforting dinners. Jeanine was the casserole queen and often shared her creations with friends and neighbors. So when Moira started to notice that her mother seemed to be losing weight, she wondered what was up. Jeanine assured Moira that she was unchanged, still shopping and cooking and doing just fine, thank you. But a few weeks later, Moira checked the pantry and refrigerator and was astounded to see it mostly empty. She and her mother started to talk more about the details of her shopping and cooking habits and Jeanine was more forthcoming. She struggled to get to the store, and she had to admit that she almost scraped another car in the store parking lot. Since then, she had become fearful of driving. And once she got home with her groceries, it just took so long to get them in the house and she was surprised how tired she was. Jeanine felt lucky if she was able to open a can of soup and heat it up for dinner, but confirmed that there were more nights she just went to bed without eating.

- Joseph, at eighty, had been a widower for several years. Like many men in this situation, he found that he was suddenly "in demand." Ladies at the senior center he attended became very attentive and he developed, with some amusement, a fairly active social life at an unexpected time. He went to concerts and lunches with his women friends and still had time for his own interests in attending city council meetings regularly. But when he developed pneumonia one winter and ended up in the hospital for a week, he found that his energy was so low on his return home that he needed help with getting around his apartment. Shopping and cooking were out of the question. The home health nurse who was sent by the hospital doctor to assess him after his hospitalization told Joseph that while he was still recovering, he needed to have some home care help.

Definition of level one: Limited time means that the number of hours in a day that a person needs a caregiver is for a few hours or part of a day, every day, or only a few days of the week. This could be a temporary or ongoing arrangement.

Level one is when your elder family member needs the following care or assistance:

- Medication management: If your mother can take her pills from a pill box with some phone call reminders from you or other family, but has difficulty organizing and setting up the pill box. Some agency care providers are not allowed to administer medications in some states. See "Who Can Give Medications at Home?"
- Bathing and dressing: Your parent can physically get into the shower with minimal help, but needs someone to be standing by for safety. For example, this is a person who has had a single fall in the past, but had a good recovery and has generally good balance.
- Meals and eating: Meal planning and preparation have become a challenge, from going to the store to cooking. This person would still love (or needs the change of scenery) to get out to the store, but needs someone to drive or accompany them. This family member might also participate in preparing food or be able to heat up a premade meal.

- Safety: Your elder family member is still able to turn off the stove when done cooking, lock the front door every night, and does not get confused and wander outside.

Types of home care to consider at this level:

- Family and nonprofessional help: If family members, friends, or neighbors are available to pitch in, this would be a good, money-saving move. A family/volunteer schedule to bring meals that can be reheated, a once-a-week shopping expedition with the elder, taking turns calling to remind to take pills, or an adult child who has time to stand by while their parent is showering and getting dressed. If it looks like a temporary situation that has an end point (a cast comes off on a specified date, a spouse returns from a trip), moving in with a family member or friend can also work well.
- Professional caregiver: Often at this level, the family may be unclear if this is going to be a permanent or a temporary arrangement. Working with a care agency can be most expedient and at the lower number of hours, perhaps not as expensive. But be forewarned: most agencies increase their hourly rate for fewer hours or have a minimum hour requirement. For example, if only one hour of time is requested, it could be billed at $30 an hour, while a four-hour shift of time is billed at $25 an hour. The care at this level can also be done with a private caregiver. One caregiver we know likes to keep her profile on Care.com regularly updated. She schedules some short-term clients as well as some part-time regular clients so that she has more flexibility and can maximize the time that she spends with her own family.
- Other options: Meals on Wheels will deliver a hot meal once a day most days of the week in many localities for those who qualify. Many catering companies offer custom meals delivered at varying prices and packages. There are devices with timers to sound alarms up to four times a day to remind someone to take prescribed medications on time. Some patients may qualify to have their doctor order a home health aide in addition to a Registered Nurse to come for brief weekly visits to assist with bathing and dressing for a temporary specified number of weeks that would be paid for by

Medicare. In some states, Medicaid may provide home care for certain patients who qualify.

Who Can Give Medications at Home?

The legalities of home care workers giving medications to their clients have been a long, ongoing debate across the country. Currently, it is legal for a home caregiver to give oral medications to their clients in twenty-nine states and the District of Columbia.[2] To determine what is allowed in your state, we recommend that you go to the following website: www.longtermscorecard.org. There you can see the state-by-state chart from the Scorecard on Long-Term Services and Supports for Older Adults, People with Physical Disabilities, and Family Caregivers, a revealing report compiled by AARP, the Commonwealth Fund, and the Scan Foundation. Whether or not it is legal in your state could change. While it may seem like a nonissue to many because family members and patients themselves have no special training and are often responsible for this task, it is a serious issue to other professionals.

Registered Nurses (RNs), for example, see their role passing meds in skilled nursing facilities and assisted living homes diminishing as this responsibility has been handed over to "medication techs" or others of a Certified Nurse Assistant (CNA) level. The reason is primarily a cost saving as the salary of an RN is obviously much higher than that of the CNA. These CNAs and others usually have a short period of training that may include a special certification that designates them as skilled at passing medications. The RN in this situation acts as the supervisor of the CNA-level professionals.

In the home, it is a different situation. There is not usually an RN or Licensed Practical Nurse (LPN) supervising the medications given on a daily basis. In those states where it is not legal for care providers to give medications to their clients, care agencies will have a professional RN or LPN come to give the medications, an added service that results in a much higher bill to the client. In privately hired caregiver scenarios, this responsibility may not even be discussed in legal terms. The task may simply be done by the caregiver and many times neither party is even aware of any illegalities.

Level Two: Regularly Scheduled Care under Twenty-Four Hours a Day

Triggers for level two:

- Anna is a divorced forty-four-year-old woman with no children. She lives with her father, James, who invited her to move in after her rent was raised beyond her means a few years ago. Anna works the evening shift at the hospital. It has been a good arrangement for both of them. While James's health has always been hardy, he was recently diagnosed with dementia. He functions quite well when Anna is with him in the daytime. However, some evenings while Anna is at work, James has become increasingly confused and anxious. Anna received a call at work from a neighbor last week when James wandered over to the neighbor's house at 9 p.m. asking if Muriel, his deceased wife, was there. After this incident, Anna started to realize that her father is fine at night when she has the weekends off and she is there with him. She often reassures him in the evenings when he starts to worry. She knows that if he had someone there to keep him company and remind him to go to bed on time, he would probably be just fine. She talks to her father's doctor, who agrees and explains that James appears to be exhibiting Sundowner's Syndrome, a symptom of dementia in which a person becomes increasingly confused or agitated as night falls and the skies darken. The doctor recommends that Anna find someone to stay with James when she is at work.
- Betty loves the retirement community where she has lived for ten years. She has always been a proactive, "take the bull by the horns" kind of person, and when her husband passed away eleven years ago, she decided to move into a smaller place. She liked the atmosphere of the retirement community that two of her best friends had moved to, so she found an apartment there for herself. After a hip replacement last July, however, she has really struggled to get up in the mornings and get herself dressed and ready to go for the day. She wakes up to horrible arthritic pain and seems to be all thumbs for the first couple of hours that she is awake. Once she does manage that awkward and time-consuming task, she is able to use her walker to get herself to the dining room for lunch and be around friends and meet her book group and even go on outings with the

community's bus service. She just wants a little help in the mornings to physically assist her when her pain is at its worst and her muscles are so slow to move.

Definition of level two: Whether it is a four-hour daily caregiver stay to help the elder get going for the day and prepare a meal for them to eat later or a person to stay overnight with someone who is fearful of being alone but fine in the daytime, this level involves a regularly scheduled caregiving service under twenty-four hours. This generally indicates an ongoing arrangement that is not expected to reverse to smaller needs, but may in fact evolve into a case for a greater number of caregiver hours.

Level two is when your elder family member needs the following care or assistance:

- Medication management: Again, home caregivers handing medications to their clients is allowed only in certain states. If you or your elderly family member finds that pills are left in the pill box and are taken haphazardly, assistance is needed every day.
- Bathing and dressing: This person has a more complex history of falls, vertigo, sustained injuries, or loss of complete range of motion or mobility, such as following a stroke. They need help with bathing and dressing in an ongoing way.
- Meals and eating: This person may or may not be able to reheat a prepared meal, but needs regular assistance with shopping and preparing fully nutritious meals.
- Safety: Advancing dementia or confusion often play a role at this level in triggering ongoing need for supervision to maintain the safety of the person and the environment. The person is forgetful of leaving doors unlocked or turning off water from the faucet and more. They may have started wandering.

Types of home care to consider at this level:

- Family: There are many family caregivers that manage the care at this level in spite of the ongoing challenges and stress. Often several generations, including the spouse, the adult children, grandchildren in their teens, and younger children take shifts caring for an elder. This is ideal when it is possible, but in our ever-changing society, not always realistic.

- Professional caregiver: This is an excellent level to do a robust search for a reliable private care agency or private hire caregiver. This situation offers both the client and the caregiver a circumstance to develop an ongoing relationship and rapport. In other words, a commitment from both parties, clear expectations of regular hours and schedule, and well-spelled-out responsibilities can result in an ideal home care outcome.
- Other: There are many technological devices coming onto the market to assist long-distance and working families to monitor their elderly family members still residing in their homes. The Nanny Cam has evolved to the Granny Cam, with some advantages and some legitimate protests for privacy and independence for adults. While there are many creative ideas emerging in technology in the senior care field, it should be considered with caution. We'll tell you about a few more of these products at the end of this chapter. These products are not at a stage that they can replace human supervision and assistance. At best, they could be considered useful temporarily or useful as a security device to monitor and prevent criminal activity of hired caregivers.

Level Three: Twenty-Four-Hour Home Care

Triggers for level three:

- For Mary, it seems like so much has changed within a short period of time, but really it simply did not get on her family's radar until after her husband passed away last spring. Mary has always been grateful for her friends, though as she grows older, their numbers are declining. Sadly, she was diagnosed with dementia this past year. She is fiercely proud and tries to continue to be active intellectually, but has medical problems that have multiplied, including osteoarthritis, a hip replacement, high blood pressure, osteoporosis, and heart failure—a combination that has impaired her walking and caused chronic pain. Until now, Mary has managed in her home that she shared for many years with her husband. Mary's husband managed all of the finances and initiated the activities that they both loved doing: going to the theater, seeing movies and lectures, and watching movies on their home DVD player. When Mary's husband died it became clear that Mary had no idea how to manage money, so her daughter, Laura, took over this task, paying all of the bills and going through all of Mary's mail and accounts to make sure all of her finances were in order. Mary's entire family was very supportive, but they live out of state. It wasn't long before Laura was coming to the house every day to do shopping and some cooking. She would respond to emergency calls from her mother when Mary would get confused in the evening, sometimes driving over and spending the night when Mary would call in a panic with pain she couldn't manage or confusion and anxiety. One night Mary wandered out her front door into the snowy street and started calling out to strangers for help, saying things like "my family wants to move me out of my home!" Fortunately, a neighbor took her in and called the daughter, averting what could have been a disaster. The situation was exhausting and was taking a toll on Laura's health and impacting her performance at work. One night Laura realized that Mary was not taking her medications correctly and that this could be contributing to the confusion and increased pain at night. She also noticed that her mother was less interested in eating and worried that Mary was not drinking enough water. There were long periods of time during the day when Mary was alone and unsupervised despite Laura's best efforts to fill in the gaps.

- Irene is proud that she has made it past her ninetieth year and still lives in her own home, thinks clearly, and has a very good memory. She has to deal with some other annoying problems though, such as being incontinent and not being able to walk without that blasted walker. Over the past three years, she has had a delightful caregiver in the daytime who helps her bathe and dress and get to appointments. In the last six months she has fallen in the middle of the night three times, each time trying to make it to the bathroom by herself (she refuses to use the bedside commode). Because of the last fall, she ended up in the hospital with a sprained back. Her longtime doctor smiled at her gently and said, "Irene, it's time that you have some overnight company."

Definition of level three: This person needs supervision for a full twenty-four hours a day. The most significant contrast with this level and the others is that your parent would be at risk of injury if left alone for more than an hour at a time, if even that. They may and probably do need some of the assistance mentioned with the previous levels, but most especially their judgment has changed to the point that they need supervision. It is also important to note that this level of care can be, but should not be, done by one individual. While many family caregivers, especially spouses, have done this 'round-the-clock care, it is generally understood that in a short period of time, it is to the detriment of their own health.

Level three is when your elder family member needs the following care or assistance:

- Medication management: There are some who can still manage to take the medications properly at this level, but it is likely that most will need prescriptions to be managed and given by someone else.
- Bathing and dressing: Due to changes in mobility, balance, and limitations in range of motion and/or judgment, the elder needs daily help in this area. These individuals will also need assistance with transferring in and out of beds, chairs, cars, and showers.
- Meals and eating: The elderly usually have a reduction in appetite as they grow older, but they continue to need a balanced and nutritious diet. Some people with stroke or motion disorders will need assistance with being fed.
- Safety: At level three, safety and security become an even bigger priority. The person's history reveals behavior or accidents that indicate that they need 'round-the-clock supervision.

Types of home care to consider at this level:

- Family: As always, families are capable of anything that they set their collective minds to do. However, we have seen so many burn out at this level. Even with large families, we have observed that the majority of the work tends to fall on one adult child over the others. Some family members may have the best of intentions, but their efforts to help the elder stay home amounts to sporadically filling in or doing one or two good deeds now and then, mostly distracted by their own busy lives and responsibilities. Meanwhile, the unmarried sibling who has been elected to move in with mom or dad struggles to manage all the needs of the aging parent. As with spouses who are the primary caregiver for their husband or wife, the adult child caregiver who goes full time often must endure fatigue, isolation, high levels of stress, and can even have a sense of not being appreciated by the rest of the family or the parent.

- Professional caregiver: We are stating the obvious here, but this is when you have more than one, in fact perhaps a group of, caregiver(s) who can take shifts throughout the week and overnight. With the home care agency, they will arrange all the shifts and find the best caregivers for your parents for you. If the night shift person is sick, they will find a substitute. With privately hired caregivers, you may need to have an extra person who is available to sub for others if they are unavailable. In the world of privately hired care, many caregivers welcome an extra shift, especially when they are already familiar with the client and their needs.

- Other: This is a level where creatively mixing and matching care may arise out of necessity or because it works out well. Perhaps a family member (unmarried sibling, college student, grandchild, or other) is available two or three nights a week to sleep over and provide supervision and safety. Some elders may participate in elder day care and spend some weekday hours with other supervision outside of their home. The best advice here is to keep the schedule as consistent as possible and have a backup plan if your elderly family member needs an urgent medical appointment or other unexpected event.

HAVING "THE TALK"

Now that you have gone through all of our levels and feel confident in knowing where you want to begin with home care, all you have to do now is convince mom or dad that this is in their best interest! There are so many variables to how you decide to approach this talk, including the nature of your relationship with your elder. Is it close? Is there conflict or geographical distance between you? Cognitive impairment, such as with Alzheimer's or other dementias, depression, or anxiety can complicate matters. Choosing the time of day is important as well. Opting for morning when you know your elder is clearer and has more energy may be better. Decide whether to include other family members in the discussion. Sometimes having another family member can be reinforcing, but other times may make the person feel "ganged up on."

- Bob is a ninety-two-year-old veteran who has had a distinguished career in the air force as a fighter pilot. He has a daughter, Jasmine, and a son, Sam. Both adult children have been supportive and involved in Bob's life. Sam's relationship with his father has been strained through the years due to disagreement on politics and Bob's opinion that Sam is "pushy" and controlling. Bob has managed to live independently in an apartment for many years, but he falls one day and breaks his leg, requiring surgery. The ensuing recovery and rehabilitation is slow and arduous, complicated by Bob's uncontrolled diabetes and heart failure. When it is time for him to be discharged from his rehabilitation center, the medical team insists that Bob will need home care help in his apartment because he still isn't able to transfer from his wheelchair safely. Bob completely balks at this idea, stating confidently that he has always taken care of himself and can do so now. Jasmine and Sam talk about how to approach their father and decide that it is best that Sam not be involved in the discussion at all. Jasmine is able to talk to her father about the short-term need for help in the home, and he finally agrees.

Accept that you may need to have a series of conversations. But before we get into the nitty gritty (and it can get gritty) about ways to approach the topic, let's begin by talking about the importance of advance directives.

Advance directives (sometimes referred to as durable power of attorney for health care) can play an important role later on, not only for the talk, but so much more. If you and your family have not completed this important document, do so, but where you are in the Home Care Needs Scale may determine how you want to approach the subject.

Advance directives are legal documents that allow you to spell out your decisions about end-of-life care ahead of time and designate a surrogate decision maker in the event that you are unable to make decisions on your own behalf. They give you a way to tell your wishes to family, friends, and healthcare professionals and to avoid confusion later. Each state has a different document and requirements for filling out the document, but essentially they all have the same purpose. Talking about the document before filling it out (most elders designate one or more children to be their healthcare power of attorney) opens up the discussion about some of the events that can indicate the need for a surrogate decision maker. For example: a medical event like a heart attack or stroke, a fall that results in a fracture of a bone requiring surgery, dehydration that requires IV fluid in the hospital, or a urinary tract infection. These discussions pave the way for honest evaluation of potential problems and solutions to those problems. If you feel comfortable, this may be a time to begin a discourse on the possibility of bringing additional care into the home after such an event. Some families even go so far as to interview care agencies in advance of any problem so they won't be scrambling later during a crisis. You could even consider finding a place on the advance directives document or add an addendum that specifies which care agency should be called during a time of need.

Assuming that you already have advance directives in place and it is time for "the talk," we have the following suggestions and tips. Always keep in mind that no one likes to have their decision-making ability taken away. As busy people, it can be tempting to rush into this process by just deciding what is best for someone without their involvement or opinion. In most cases this is a huge mistake. Most people like to have control over their environment and decisions and there are ways to honor this while gently guiding someone.

- Be aware of and acknowledge your own feelings before beginning: You have a history with your family that is unique and complicated. This history may be characterized by unresolved conflict or disagreements, family dynamics that favor one child over another, guilt, or the perception of unmet expectations, to name a few. Add to that the stress and possible fear of confrontation about a subject that may bring up these feelings. You may feel anger or resentment about being placed in this position of responsibility and have stresses of your own to deal with.
- Take a tone of respect and avoid ageist expressions: Don't use condescending or degrading language. In your mind you may be thinking "my mom changed my diapers for me when I was a baby, so now I am doing the same for her." The obvious difference, regardless of how much your mother has declined, is that she is still an adult. Be respectful in both tone and attitude and use empowering and positive language, such as "you are a strong and capable person and we just want you to be as independent as possible."

Becca Levy, an associate professor of epidemiology and psychology at the Yale School of Public Health, has compiled numerous studies that show that negative stereotypes of old age can lead to worse health outcomes.[3] On the flip side, people with positive age stereotypes tend to be more likely to engage in preventative health behaviors.[4]

- Ask for support from the medical team: The elder's medical team may be a trusted primary care physician, nurse, or social worker that can help advocate for the need for help at home. We have observed physicians normalizing this suggestion by talking about other patients who have benefitted from additional help at home or even placing the suggestion in a personal context by stating, "this is what I would tell my mother if she was in your situation." For example: mom has fallen and broken her hip and has just had a hip replacement. In the rehabilitation setting she doesn't progress as quickly as she needs to and her insurance benefits are going to run out. This is the perfect time to have a private discussion with the physician about recommending home care and home health care to continue her rehabilitation at home. A person of authority can have a greater impact. Ask the physician to write an "order" for home care upon returning home. Another example: a daughter notices that dad is not taking as good care of himself as she is as accustomed to seeing. Her father has always been a dapper man, dressing with care and taking daily showers. She notices that his clothes are looking rumpled and dirty, that he smells a little bit, and that his house is more cluttered and disorganized. There may be a reasonable medical explanation like a urinary tract infection or dehydration. Now may be the perfect time to suggest a trip to his primary care physician to rule out a reversible condition by requesting a complete medical evaluation. Meanwhile, make a call to the physician's office and speak with the nurse to explain the problem and ask that the doctor make a recommendation of home care during the visit if he or she thinks this is a reasonable suggestion.
- Be honest: Honesty is part of respect. Be authentic and open about what you observe the problems to be and do so without trying to elicit guilt.

- Anticipate objections in advance: Anticipating what objections might arise in advance will make it easier to respond in a calm manner without getting defensive.
- Deal with denial: Denial can be a powerful obstacle to the idea of bringing in home care help. By denial we mean a person's refusal to acknowledge that they need any assistance. It can be challenging to assess the cause of this. In cases in which people already have some cognitive impairment or diagnosed dementia, this is expected, because people lose their awareness of their abilities or may even forget that they have problems! One solution might be to write down the specific tasks the elder is having difficulty with so these can be referred back to later. In the end, you can't make someone do what they do not want to do. Depending on the circumstances, you may take the chance of just introducing someone as if this was planned all along. Be prepared for this to backfire, however, and be ready to jettison the idea if necessary moving forward. However, we have seen elders with complete command of all their faculties deny even the most obvious disabilities. In this instance, it may take a team approach using other family members, physicians, and friends to gently point out obvious safety concerns.
- Negotiate: Most of us want to make our own decisions, and as your elder begins to lose independence, this becomes even more important. The small losses in someone's life may not seem that important to you, but try putting yourself in your elder's shoes. What would it feel like to have someone question your ability to drive or make decisions for yourself? Finding a way to empower that person can make the process go more smoothly. Try negotiating by asking for a compromise that can be revisited at a later designated date or "agree to disagree," recognizing the value of opposing opinions while looking for a solution to the problem that everyone can accept or at least try. For example, suggest that a caregiver come in on a trial basis (perhaps with less time than you have in mind) to be evaluated, and if your elder doesn't like the caregiver or the presence of someone in the house, then you agree to discontinue. If you can hand pick a good caregiver, then chances are things will go well.
- Be specific: Instead of using vague expressions like "dad, we don't think you are doing well," use specific examples of safety concerns,

such as pointing out that dad is leaving the stove on after cooking, there is evidence that medications are not being taken correctly, falls or difficulty with walking and balance have been observed, or there is no food in the fridge, indicating that nutrition could be an issue. Genuinely express your concerns in the context of safety and security.

THE COST OF CARE: SOMETIMES IT TAKES A VILLAGE

The cost of home care is an expensive proposition. While a certain amount of help for part of the day may be manageable and less costly than moving into assisted living, the price soars with 'round-the-clock care or anything close to twenty-four-hour care. Before panicking, research the possibility of your elder qualifying for state-sponsored assistance or other support in the home. Consider these nuts-and-bolts ideas, as well as additional creative cost solutions, in chapter 9.

Each state will have different programs and criteria, and here are some possible options to explore:

- The most expedient way to see if a family member may benefit from state-supported caregiver resources is to access Eldercarelocator.gov. This is a public service provided by the U.S. Administration on Aging that provides grants to states to fund a wide range of supports to assist family caregivers, including respite and caregiver training.
- If your elder is a veteran, he or she may qualify for financial assistance through a program called Aid and Attendance. Call your local Veteran's Administration for more information about the criteria for qualification.
- Look to your church or faith group for possible caregiver programs that may offer assistance. For example, Jewish Family Services provides support for older adults in many states. These services may include respite care to family caregivers and some day services.
- Check on your elder's possible eligibility for the Medicaid waiver program. These programs vary state by state, but provide services in the home in lieu of nursing home care.

- Income and asset qualifications are stringent. Over time, state governments have observed that keeping an elder in the home or assisted living with help is more cost effective than paying for nursing home care. If your elder's financial situation is complicated and you are unsure about Medicaid eligibility, you may want to consider hiring an estate planning attorney who is familiar with your state's Medicaid law.

MORE DETAILS ABOUT MEDICAID COVERAGE

Can Medicaid in your state help with the cost of home care? Medicaid is a federally funded health insurance program for people with low income and few assets. In all states, Medicaid provides coverage for some low-income people, families and children, pregnant women, the elderly, and people with disabilities. In some states, Medicaid has been expanded to cover all adults below a certain income level. Medicaid programs must follow federal guidelines, but coverage and costs may be different from state to state. Some Medicaid programs pay for your care directly. Others use private insurance companies to provide Medicaid coverage. Not all nursing homes accept Medicaid, so you need to check to make certain that Medicaid is accepted as a payer source.

Unlike Medicare coverage of home health care or regular Medicaid long-term care nursing home coverage, Medicaid waiver programs aren't limited to medical care and their coverage doesn't run out when a person's medical condition stabilizes. The purpose of these waiver programs is to keep people out of nursing homes for as long as possible because nursing home care is more expensive than providing support in a home-based setting. The median cost of a nursing home in 2016 is $6,844 for a semi-private room[5] and the median cost for home care based on forty-four hours a week is $3,813 a month.[6] These costs will most likely go up. Some states provide services in the home and other states will use Medicaid to support someone in assisted living.

Home and community-based services through the waiver programs can provide:

- In-home health care, including nursing care and physical therapy.

- Home care services to help with the normal activities of daily living (ADLs), such as eating, bathing, and dressing.
- Homemaker services, such as simple cooking, cleaning, and laundry.
- Meal delivery.
- Adult day services participation (care, companionship, and activities at an adult day services center).
- Transportation assistance to and from medical care or other services.
- Assistive devices, medical equipment, and supplies.
- Minor home modifications (such as widening a doorway to accommodate a wheelchair or installing a safety railing in a bathtub).

To give a state-specific example of Medicaid eligibility, in California an individual must have below $2,000 in assets and make less than a $16,395 year to qualify.[7] Some individuals choose to "spend down" their assets in order to qualify for Medicaid, but even if they qualify for Medicaid, that doesn't necessarily mean a nursing home will accept them. They must also meet the criteria for nursing home placement, meaning they are unable to take care of themselves at home. Regardless of the state you live in, consult an attorney who specializes in Medicaid eligibility or your local Area Agency on Aging to inquire about Medicaid waiver programs as a possible way to help support your elder at home.

If all else fails, it will be time to make a serious assessment of the costs of providing care now and for the future. Many families are shocked to find out that Medicare doesn't pay for home care or for long-term care in a nursing home (see table 2.1). Medicare only pays for rehabilitation after a three-night stay in the hospital, and depending on the type of Medicare insurance, the rehabilitation services are only paid up to twenty days. After that the individual may be responsible for the per day rate to stay in rehab unless they have secondary insurance to pay for up to one hundred days.

Adding to the stress of these considerations is the fact that discussions between generations about finances can be awkward and seen as an intrusion on one's privacy. Also, there may be differences in the ability of various family members to contribute to the cost of care, which can lead to resentment and frustration. Family members may be in far better shape financially to contribute to care than the elder themself. The cost of home care can seem outrageous to an elder who has been independent and thrifty their entire life and plans on leaving savings and other assets to their children.

- Nancy is an eighty-eight-year-old woman who prided herself on being conservative with money and not making unnecessary purchases. Her husband, James, died last year and she is left in the home they bought twenty-two years ago. She is startled to find out that their home is not paid for and there is a remaining mortgage. Nancy had always left the house payments to James and now she is thrust into the role of having to take on these tasks. Nancy has also had increasing pain related to spinal stenosis and osteoporosis, making it increasingly difficult to manage a home where James took on many of these responsibilities. Nancy loves her home and the garden out back where she grows flowers and sits to listen to the birds sing, but she is feeling overwhelmed. Nancy's children suggest assisted living, but Nancy is adamant about remaining in her home. One of Nancy's daughters, Jan, asks to become Nancy's financial power of attorney so she can evaluate the bills and accounts. Jan discovers that there is a small retirement account of about $50,000 and James's social security income of $1,750 and that is all there is, not leaving Nancy enough to pay for home care and too much to qualify for Medicaid. Jan and her siblings are willing to contribute some, but don't want to jeopardize their own financial security, and no one is in favor of tapping into Nancy's limited savings. Jan decides to consult her bank and finds out that Nancy can take out a reverse mortgage, which will provide enough income to pay for the home care and leave the remaining equity in the home to Nancy's children. (This is only an illustration. Requirements and criteria for reverse mortgages and home equity lines of credit vary depending on where you live and the housing market in your area.)

Doing a complete financial evaluation of all assets available to help pay for care is a good start, but keep in mind that care needs may increase to the point that it makes more fiscal sense to consider assisted living. A good, reputable estate planning attorney can put together short- and long-range plans.

Families often find themselves in a quandary about how to broach the topic of assisted living considering the costs of home care in someone's home. Quite frankly, many elders want to remain in their homes and should have the opportunity to do so.

- George is an eighty-six-year-old man who was receiving seven hours a day of home care after he became ill with a bacterial infection that sapped his strength and energy, leaving him unable to cook, clean, bathe, or shop safely during the day. His children all live out of state. Home care is costing the family $4,900 a month— enough to pay for a small, home-based assisted living where George would be safe and all of his needs would be taken care of. But there is a problem. George does not want to move from his home. So the family hires a geriatric care manager to look at other options to keep George in his home. Considering that George was doing fine before he became ill, the family is hoping that with time he will need less care and not more. The geriatric care manager finds a senior center close by that will pick George up and bring him home. She arranges to take George to the senior center and have lunch. He is reluctant at first, but finds that there is a group that plays cards after lunch. George decides to give it a try. Now, for three days a week, three hours a day, he is in a safe environment and gets one meal a day while enjoying the social aspect of playing cards and meeting other people. George's wife died two years ago, and much to his surprise and delight, several women take an interest in spending time with him. The savings on home care comes to almost $1,000 a month.

Consider other "out of the box" ideas, such as finding a roommate that is more able and that can help in sharing in household duties, or perhaps a grown grandchild who needs temporary housing and can help an elder with household tasks while the elder is recovering from surgery or an illness, as mentioned in the Home Care Needs Scale. Some larger cities have "villages" where groups of elders live independently and share resources like shopping, medical appointments, and social services that are provided by volunteers. We'll talk about more of these ideas that center on pooling resources and creative financing in chapter 9.

In summary, here are the steps to take before, during, and after planning on how to pay for the cost of home care.

- Families must communicate with each other and uncover all of the available assets before discussing a plan.
- Find out if Medicaid or other income-based supports are an option. Start with your Area Agency on Aging. The Area Agency on Aging will also have information about caregiver support programs that may not have an income eligibility requirement.
- Look to faith-based programs that may offer in-home support.
- Get a good financial advisor in the banking sector or a private elder law attorney who specializes in estate planning. If there are questions about Medicaid eligibility, make sure that the estate planning person you select has experience in that area.
- Make a five-year plan with financial advice. Devise different scenarios that cover a wide range of care requirements from minimal in-home care to assisted living and residence in a long-term-care nursing home. Review the plan with your family and the elder on a regular basis.

OTHER OPTIONS TO CONSIDER

Consider the use of some of the technological advances that assist with helping family members track how elders are doing. (We have no affiliation with any of these companies and our mention of them in this section does not suggest any liability on our part. We recommend looking online for additional technological supports that are currently being developed.) There are the low-tech options like a basic emergency response system (ERS). This is typically a watch or pendant that can be pushed during an emergency that calls 911. The biggest problem with ERS devices is that elders forget to wear them or take them off and don't put them back on. Another low-tech option if someone else is living in the home with the elder is a baby monitor in the bedroom to hear if there is a problem or fall. Other more advanced fall detectors include those built into phones or other devices that can be clipped to a keychain or purse. Higher-tech options include the following:

- Companionship and healthcare monitoring such as GeriJoy and Reminder Rosie. GeriJoy utilizes remote caregivers who interface with elders via an electronic pad that uses avatars to communicate. Reminder Rosie records appointments in a family member's voice and communicates those appointments or reminders to take medications via a clock.
- GPS systems built into shoes can monitor if someone has wandered and where they go. GPS SHOE sends a signal to a central monitoring system so that the person can be tracked via website.
- Medication adherence and dispenser systems manage and monitor medication compliance. MED-E-LERT is a locking medication device that sounds an alarm when it is time to take medications. There are also systems that link with your smartphone to alert you when your parent has not taken scheduled pills from a smart dispenser.
- Environment sensors/passive monitoring system products can check a number of items within a house: motion patterns, stove on/off status, carbon dioxide or carbon monoxide levels, presence of smoke, air quality, humidity, and fire. They can dim lights remotely and lock or unlock doors. Motion sensor products can be used solely for monitoring through algorithms to automatically detect movement aberrations and reliably generate appropriate alarms. With the elder's consent, some assisted living communities use motion sensors in a person's apartment at the bathroom door alerting the staff if the bathroom door is closed and not reopened for a long period of time. The bathroom is one of the most dangerous places for an elder to have a fall or medical event. Check out Vivint, ADT, and Frontpoint.
- Home monitoring systems operate on strategically placed sensors, from motion detectors to leak or flood detectors to item-specific detectors on doors, beds, toilets, chairs, etc. You can monitor someone's daily activities and, more importantly, receive notifications when the system senses a disruption. These notifications can come to a smartphone, tablet, or computer. Some even include engagement and communications features, like text message, e-mail, or phone reminders and alerts that allow you to check in and communicate from wherever you both are. Try Quietcare, GrandCareSystems, or BeClose.

- Traditional personal emergency response systems (PERS), as mentioned previously, send alarms notifying caregivers about a fall, health emergency, home invasion, fire, or even egress/exits due to wandering. Most will also send help immediately, even if the individual can't communicate a need for assistance. There are standard one-button versions and ones with automatic fall detection capabilities. Look at Lifeline or LifeStation.
- Mobile PERS provide peace of mind on the go with models that you can take with you. Consider Mobile Help, which is a pendant that travels with the individual. If they fall or have a medical emergency, they push the button on the device and emergency responders in the area are notified. There is also the GreatCall 5Star Responder Service, which does everything from detecting falls, allowing you to make calls to emergency responders, and receiving medication reminders.
- GPS tracking systems can alert the authorities and help locate a missing person quickly. Most of these systems operate by signal exchanges from satellites and nearby cell towers when the person is traveling or wandering. The program then measures the distance between the device itself and the cell towers and satellite signals, pinpointing the individual's location and communicating this information back to the system. Try Adiant Mobile or the Alzheimer's Association Comfort Zone.
- Video monitoring can provide feedback on an elder in their home and provides direct feedback to a family member or caregiver on a smartphone, tablet, or the web.

Technology advances that help elders stay safe, connected, stimulated, and engaged in their own health and well-being continue to accelerate rapidly. Before investing in any of these, however, it is wise to do research on the companies and try to get consumer feedback on reliability, usability, and customer service support.

While these new innovations have advantages, there are several caveats. Personal privacy is often compromised and they still rely on family members' availability to manage, monitor, and supervise the environment and the information being provided. Do you realistically have the time to do this? The multitasking demands of our lives are already on overload and although it is tempting to view these technologies as alternatives to hiring someone, they too have inherent weaknesses. We hope that the future of these systems will eventually offer true relief and safety for families, but at present, it would be a mistake to rely on them completely. More tech options are discussed in chapter 5.

TAKEAWAY POINTS FOR THIS CHAPTER

- Start by becoming familiar with some key home care terms so that you can avoid confusion later on.
- Use our Home Care Needs Scale to figure out where your elder is in terms of medication management, bathing and dressing, meals and eating, and safety, and how much time they need someone else to be in the home with them.
- Approach your plan with flexibility and creativity.
- Plan for having "the talk" and realistically approach your family with the idea that it will be a series of conversations about home care solutions. Use our suggestions for making "the talk" a win-win over time for everyone involved.
- Use the advance directive as a tool for planning and communicating what your elder family member most wants.

3

FINDING THE RIGHT HIRED CAREGIVER
FOR YOU AND YOUR FAMILY

Most elders and their families have only a vague familiarity with the world of caregiving. If and when they do think about caregiving, their thoughts usually drift back a generation. What did we do when grandma was starting to need a little help? The memories usually include a family caregiver, such as an aunt who had been a homemaker and did not have a commitment to an out-of-home job. She lived very close by in the same community, had the flexible schedule to make daily visits, do the shopping, cooking, and bathing, and, most importantly, to be grandma's honored companion. If things got more complicated than that, say if grandma could no longer afford to live in her home, a family member usually took her into their home in her same loved and familiar town to remain until the end of her life. Or if grandma's health deteriorated, she may have gone to a hospital and maybe on to a nursing home to live out her last brief days.

However, things have changed since grandma's time. With medical advances, a changing healthcare system, and greater public awareness and demand for autonomy and choice at the end of life, the scene is quite different today. Not only do we have ever-increasing numbers of people over the age of sixty-five, we also have a revolution going on in how people in this country receive medical care. The older adult is uniquely impacted by this. They are increasingly more informed as consumers of health care who decide for themselves how to proceed with their care and end of life. Part and parcel with these efforts to decide for themselves is the growing choice of seniors to remain at home.

When seniors need help in their daily lives to age at home these days, it often requires more help than the family can provide. Even if there is someone in the extended family who has the time and flexibility to be a family caregiver, they may have to relocate to a different town or state to help out. Some families consider moving the elderly parent to a different state to be closer to a son or daughter who can help. We have seen mixed results with this strategy: some elders have the resilience to take in a new community with optimism and others go into a quick decline. One widowed senior we know moved from what she thought of as a lonely existence in Los Angeles after her husband died to live with her son and his family in Salt Lake City. While she had been convinced that her life had been sad and lonely in LA, she found Salt Lake City utterly boring in contrast and moved back within six months. "This place just isn't me!" When these options do not pan out, families turn to the alternatives. Hiring a professional caregiver can be daunting for the beginner. It helps to start with the basics: learning who they are, what their training is, and where to find them.

SORTING THROUGH AN ALPHABET OF CERTIFICATIONS

Clients and family members often refer to caregivers as "companions," "friends," "helpers," and "aides." Who is this person and what is truly important? Is it personality, attitude, training? The answers to these questions depend entirely on the person being helped and what they want and need. A caregiver with a great personality and attitude can bring joy and an immeasurable improvement to an elder's quality of life, but is it enough?

The lexicon of hired caregivers is confusing and complicated. Understanding the differences in training and the terminology that accompanies that training will help you make better choices. And everything depends on what state you live in. States vary significantly on what they require for training for both CNAs (Certified Nursing Assistants) and PCAs (Personal Care Assistants), along with the kinds of tasks they can perform. To give an example of two very different state requirements, let's examine the State of New York. Before an individual can even sit for the Certified Nursing Assistant Exam, they must meet the following criteria:

- Criminal background check
- Physical exam
- Tuberculosis screening
- Drug test

After meeting these criteria, an individual must have one hundred hours of training, seventy-five of which are in the classroom and then hours in an actual medical environment like an assisted living or nursing home. Then the individual can take the state exam.

In contrast, in the state of Ohio, an individual who wants to become a CNA must have seventy-five hours of a combination of classroom and clinical training. Then they sit for the exam. That's it. If you live in a state where requirements are minimal, it can be even more critical to find out what ongoing training the agency itself offers.[1] Now that you know what is required of the person that will be providing the most intimate and important care for your elder, consider what is required of your hairdresser. In New York and many other states, your hairdresser must obtain a cosmetology license by completing a *one-thousand-hour course* of study and pass the New York written and practical exam.[2] This is not to disparage hairdressers. Mandating this level of study and commitment is beneficial to the customer's safety and welfare. Why isn't the same requirement made of the people who will be caring for the most vulnerable among us?

Once you have information about training requirements under your belt, you are probably feeling well prepared to hire someone from an agency that provides good training. But training to do what exactly?

Regulations can vary widely from state to state and will define the scope of what a CNA can do. Table 3.1 is an example of two states and the differences in what CNAs are allowed to do.[3]

Certainly there are many other tasks that CNAs can perform that are worthwhile and helpful, such as help with bathing, dressing, cooking, cleaning, medication reminders (if they are not allowed by the state to actually administer the medications), transportation, and companionship. If your elder needs more medically oriented care and your state does not allow CNAs to perform those duties, you may need to look into Medicare-covered home health services, which are time limited, or hiring a

Table 3.1. What Tasks Will States Allow CNAs to Perform?

Alaska allows its CNAs to do the following medically oriented tasks:	Connecticut allows its CNAs to do the following medically oriented tasks:
• Administer glucometer test • Administer oral medication • Administer medication on an as-needed basis • Administer medication via pre-filled insulin or insulin pen • Draw up insulin for dosage requirements • Administer intramuscular medications • Administer medications through tubes • Insert suppositories	• Administer glucometer test

Source: *Raising Expectations: AARP State Scorecard on Long Term Services and Supports for Older Adults, People with Disabilities, and Family Caregivers,* 2014.

private nurse, which can be quite expensive. If you opt to hire privately, these state-by-state agency requirements are not applicable.

PERSONAL CARE AIDES

Personal care aides do not have any type of certification, and training requirements again vary from state to state. "Outdated training curricula fail to provide workers with the skills and competencies they need to deliver person-centered care in the community without the benefit of on-site supervision or support. Federal training requirements are outdated and do not reflect skills and competencies that address the complex needs of today's older and frailer consumers."[4]

Knowing the disparity among states and the minimal training requirements for PCAs regardless of state requirements behooves consumers of these services to ask questions about a particular agency's training. So for example, Utah requires six hours of training per year for PCAs. A home care company called Danville Senior Support Services in Utah requires their caregivers to complete many more hours than the minimal state requirements. This is but one example of one home care company. This may give you an idea of the type of training to ask about when considering an agency. The following training sessions at Danville are offered to PCAs, CNAs, families, and professionals:

- Diabetes: Nutrition, Exercise, Precautions, and Equipment
- Communication with People with Disabilities: Body Language/ Tone/Voice/Sign Language/Written Communication
- Muscular and Macular Degeneration
- Use of Different Equipment: Colostomy Bag and Catheter Care, Adaptive Utensils, Walkers, Braces, Bathing Chair
- Personal Care: Bathing, Dressing, Toileting
- Cooking and Meal Preparation: Nutrition, Menu Planning, Following a Recipe, Cooking, Presentation, and Encouraging Eating
- The Ultimate Housekeeper: What Clients Want, Where to Start, Where to Finish, Proper Equipment, Finishing Touches
- Helping Clients Regain Their Independence: Prompting, Reinforcement, Encouraging, Exercises, Encouraging Independence
- Assisting with Eating and Swallowing
- Comfort, Stimulation, and Quality of Life
- End of Life: Hospice, Comfort Care, Signs the End Is Near, Procedures When a Client Dies

But a word of caution: the best-trained caregiver may not be a good fit for your elder. Or an even bigger concern, what do you do if your elder has several personal care needs like bathing, dressing, medication reminders or administration, or transferring and the agency does not have a CNA available? In a perfect world you would have the option of hiring a CNA who is also a great fit, but too often it is more complicated than that. There are no easy answers to these perplexing questions, but being informed and taking the time to ask some important questions will help avoid problems later. Questions to ask include:

- Ask the agency you are thinking about hiring what their CNAs and personal care aides can do and can't do in your state. It may be necessary for you to fill in care gaps with other skilled nursing care covered under Medicare or other insurance.
- Find out what your state requires for CNAs.
- If you are not satisfied or have questions about the information you are given by a particular agency, look online to identify the tasks a CNA can do in your state and whether Personal Care Assistants have any training requirements at all.

- Ask an agency for a yearly schedule of the staff training offerings that go above and beyond state requirements.

You probably have a visual picture in your mind about who the caregiver is that you want to hire. It is human nature to expect and want the best for our aging parents. This imagined caregiver is bright, optimistic, caring, responsible, and committed to doing the best job possible. These caregivers do exist, but taking a look at the specifics of the caregiving industry will temper your expectations and give you a realistic view with which to make decisions.

The home care business is a growth industry. The Bureau of Labor Statistics projects the demand for home care aides to increase by nearly 26 percent by 2022.[5] In a joint study by the National Alliance for Caregiving and the AARP Public Policy Institute, it was found that there are over 34.2 million American adults serving as unpaid caregivers to someone aged fifty or older. Six in ten caregivers care for an adult with a long-term physical condition and one-quarter indicate the person they care for has a memory problem. In the same study, 78 percent of caregivers reported the need for more information and help with caregiving topics.[6] The Paraprofessional Healthcare Institute reports that personal and home health aides are projected to be the fastest growing occupations in the country, increasing by 71 percent and 69 percent respectively until 2020.[7] The *New York Times* reports, "Topping the list of occupations expected to grow between 2012 and 2022 are personal care aides, in the No. 1 slot (580,800 new positions); home health aides, No. 4 (424,200 jobs); and nursing assistants, No. 6 (312,200 jobs)."[8]

Now pair those eye-opening statistics with a rapidly aging population. Between 2012 and 2060, the United States will experience considerable growth in its older population. In 2060, the population aged sixty-five and over is projected to be 83.7 million, almost double its estimated population of 43.1 million in 2012. The baby boomers are largely responsible for this increase in the older population, as they began turning sixty-five in 2011.[9]

You are obviously not alone in your quest to find a good caregiver for your elder. Considering what a significant growth industry this is, one might assume that workers would be attracted to these positions. A closer examination reveals why there is a constant and troubling shortage of private duty caregivers. According to the Bureau of Labor Statistics, the mean hourly wage for caregivers is $10.48 an hour. Eighty-five percent of caregivers are women and nearly 50 percent are people of color.[10] Although many agencies do not offer benefits, they are now required to pay overtime and offer health insurance if they meet the federal employee requirement. Moreover, as of this writing, two states, California and New York, have passed legislation mandating minimum wage of $15.00 an hour. This is great news for caregivers, but how will this affect consumers? Academics like Ai-Jen Poo in her book *The Age of Dignity: Preparing for the Elder Boom in a Changing America* are looking at creative approaches using state and federal resources to supplement the care of elders at home.

In light of these rather sobering statistics, what are the real lives of these caregivers? Why do they choose this profession considering the poverty wages, lack of job security, and difficulty of the work? Is there any wonder that there is a high turnover in this business?

CAREGIVER INTERVIEW

Sherry has been in the private duty business for over thirty-five years, starting when she was in high school. She began with a maid service that evolved into providing personal tasks for clients. The Certified Nursing Assistant designation did not exist when she started this work. As the years went by, small agencies bought larger ones and Sherry worked for one agency after the other. She has been with her current agency for thirteen years and says: "I am the employee with the most time with the agency. During our staff meetings, most caregivers when introduced state they have been with the agency for a month, or sometimes a year, but rarely longer. It is a revolving door."

Here are some of the questions I asked Sherry:

Why are you doing this work?

I love working with the elderly. I used to have my CNA license, but I let it lapse because with a CNA license you get placed with people who only need personal care like bathing and I prefer the companionship side of the business.

What is the hardest part of this job?

Losing someone. Being pulled from a client to work with another one when you have been working with someone for a long time. Also the driving from client to client! I have seen many changes in this industry, mostly that there are many more immigrants working at the company, which is not a bad thing, but many of them are unskilled at even simple tasks like making a bed and their grasp of English is very poor. I also feel badly for some clients who have multiple caregivers coming in all the time.

What would you like to see changed about your working conditions?

Higher pay! The company I work for has decent pay and benefits and they have regular training. As an incentive for attending trainings we get gift cards and credit toward levels within the company. I am at the Gold level, which gives me paid time off. I have attended all the offered trainings and have not been late for work.

How many of your clients over the last few years have had dementia?

Most of them. I feel that I can handle most situations with clients with dementia, but there have been a handful that have been difficult.

Why not work in an assisted living facility where the hours would be steady and you wouldn't have to drive so much?

I have never liked the structure of assisted living where people are told what do and when to do it. I prefer the atmosphere of someone's home where clients can do what they want when they want. It's not as if I let someone sleep all day if they want to when I know it isn't good for them, but there is more flexibility in someone's home.

SPECIAL CARE DESIGNED FOR SPECIAL CARE NEEDS

According to the Alzheimer's Association, 37 percent of people aged eighty-five and over have Alzheimer's or other related dementia disorders. Forty-four percent of people age seventy-five to eighty-four have Alzheimer's or related dementias. And these are just the folks that have been diagnosed.[11] Training and preparation to work with elders with dementia would seem to be a logical piece of the private duty system.

"Direct-care workers have difficult jobs, and they may not receive the training necessary to provide dementia care. One review found that direct-care workers received, on average, 75 hours of training and that this training included little focus on issues specific or pertinent to dementia care. Turnover rates are high among direct-care workers, and recruitment and retention are persistent challenges."[12]

It is more likely than not that if you are looking to hire a caregiver for an elder, that person has some signs of dementia that can require a unique set of skills to manage. Can your caregiver handle someone with dementia?

The 2016 Alzheimer's Disease Facts and Figures outlines some of the symptoms that a caregiver will need to manage to provide care to an elder with dementia:

- Wandering, especially at night
- Depressed mood
- Anxiety
- Agitation and sometimes even aggression
- Inappropriate behavior such as sexual acting out
- Poor judgment, which can lead to safety concerns (an example: going downstairs, attempting to cook or drive)
- Inability to remember simple instructions

Ask the agency or online service you are considering hiring whether they provide dementia-specific training and what that training consists of.

HOW TO HIRE: HIRING PRIVATELY, THROUGH AN AGENCY, AND A WHOLE NEW WORLD OF ONLINE CHOICES

The basic rundown of the four primary avenues to hiring a professional caregiver are outlined in table 3.2. We will explore more about each in this section.

THE CLASSIC PRIVATE HIRE

Before our discussion comparing what type of agency or online alternatives are now available for finding good caregivers for your family, we need to talk about the more informal word of mouth private hiring that still takes place. This is the classic form of privately hiring caregivers that

Table 3.2.   Four Ways to Hire a Caregiver

Classic: Hire Privately	Traditional: "Brick and Mortar" Care Agency	Freelance Style: Internet-Based Company	Hybrid: Online-Based Care Agencies
Friends, acquaintances, or a caregiver that you already know refer you to good caregivers.	A doctor, nurse, or hospital suggests several agencies that they know that have helped patients of theirs. These companies have brochures in doctor's offices and local and national advertising. The agency is the employer and typically offers low wages and hours and no benefits.	Caregivers and families find each other on these sites. Caregivers are not the employee of the company, but are freelance employees who register their services there. Families can read caregiver profiles and compare with other caregivers.	Consumers register online with the agency and can view and choose caregivers in online profiles. Caregivers are the employees of the online agency, not the consumer. These agencies typically offer higher salaries and some benefits and training to maintain a higher standard of care and employee retention.
Pros: Seemingly simple and less expensive, but requires the same diligent verification as a third-party employer. *Cons:* You can be lulled into trusting an applicant without fully vetting them.	*Pros:* The professional association with the medical community enhances the reputation of the agency. *Cons:* Traditional agencies have high turnover of employees, sometimes leading to inconsistent care of elders.	*Pros:* Consumers have more control of choice of caregivers. Salaries are negotiable. Caregivers can choose who they want to work for and typically have a higher rate of pay and job stability. *Cons:* Consumers have greater responsibility for payroll, insurance, and other additional liability for employees.	*Pros:* Consumers do not have the added responsibility of doing background checks, payroll, taxes, and insurance. Some of these online marketplace care agencies have a flat rate listed directly on the site, making the costs more transparent. *Cons:* It is not clear how effective direct supervision of the caregivers is in comparison to a traditional care agency.

has existed for many generations. You mention that you are looking for someone to help your mother-in-law who needs some help with personal care. A friend knows another friend whose father had the most capable and caring person who is a retired nurse and she happens to be available. Or a co-worker has a neighbor who just passed away and she had a great caregiver and your co-worker can give you his or her number. These personal referrals seem to be made of gold because of the people that you know who bring them to your attention. Of course, you trust your friend or co-worker. The referral may in fact be the best caregiver in the world. But it is imperative that you do all the steps to verify the potential employee before hiring them as you would do in any other situation. When you are not hiring through an agency, to protect your family, *you must:*

1. Do a background check and drug screening.
2. Confirm credentials such as the CNA or training as a Personal Care Assistant.
3. Verify previous employment.
4. Get references other than the person you have in common.

If you have never done any of these actions before, please read the section "Hiring Privately? Don't Skimp on Verification!" *with suggestions on how to accomplish them.*

This may feel awkward if you are concerned about offending your friend or co-worker who made the recommendation. Perhaps you worry that you will offend the caregiver and they are in such demand that they will go find another family who won't bother them with such details. Get over it! In this day and age, if a caregiver does not know how important verification is to their own reputation, they are probably not who you are looking for.

Many personal referrals are known for a limited time and may indeed have been good employees. Some people who are hired informally may have no training or certification. While we strongly recommend hiring people with certification, when hiring privately, it is your choice. You do want clarification of this as part of your hiring decision to get an accurate picture of the applicant's experience with specific care activities. In other situations, an applicant may have a criminal history that your friend may be unaware of. They may have a problem with drug abuse that is not apparent on the surface. These are all red flags that if ignored can have grave consequences for the safety and security of your loved ones.

HIRING PRIVATELY? DON'T SKIMP ON VERIFICATION!

- Background checks: Background checks require that you inform the applicant that you are doing a background check and receive their written permission to do so.[13] The standard is to look back on the record for the past six or seven years.[14] If your potential employee is registered on Care.com, as many freelance caregivers are, it may be easiest and quickest to purchase the background check there. (Some caregivers on Care.com[15] have earned CarePro Badges and you can see their background check on their profile, without added cost to you.) You can ask the applicant to request their own current Identity History Summary Report through the FBI's Criminal Justice Information Services[16] at https://www.fbi.gov/about-us/cjis/identity-history-summary-checks for about $18. They can get the report themselves and bring it to you. However, this process is complicated and can take months! There are private companies that are deemed official FBI channelers by the FBI, such as My FBI Report,[17] that can obtain the FBI report of an individual more quickly for a bigger fee. This fee may be worth it to you or your applicant to expedite this vital task. Depending on your state and the online court system, you can look up an individual by name in the different counties and court levels of a jurisdiction (for example, civil or circuit) and check the record for free. This method is useful if employment records confirm that the person has lived in the same locale for many years. There are background screening services online, but our experience is that they may not all be very reliable.
- Drug screening: Drug screening should be considered an essential tool to give you the most current picture of your applicant's status. Many instacare-type medical facilities offer walk-in drug testing for a nominal fee. The applicant must of course sign to share the results with you so that you can get them from the facility independently of the caregiver applicant. If there is any hemming and hawing about why they can't get to the drug screening in a timely manner, you will want to move on to the next applicant. Remember, drug screening should be an ongoing

tool for your employees and you can explain when they are hired that random drug screening will be a part of their employment.

- Confirm credentials: Ask the applicant to bring you a copy of his or her most recent CNA license or other certification. If someone has let this lapse due to financial constraints and they can show you their dated certification, that may suffice depending on your circumstances.
- Verify past employment: This is usually a simple matter of getting a list of past employers and their phone numbers and calling them to confirm that the applicant has indeed been employed there.
- Get references: After hearing a glowing report from your friend or co-worker, this can seem like one you can skip. But remember, the more people that you connect with that establish the applicant is really who they say they are, the better. David Petroski, owner of Grandma Joan's Live-In Care Service (http://www.grandmajoans.net/), asserts that he values references highly. While his company does criminal background checks too, he finds that the information that he gets from a caregiver's references are very revealing and informative. He advises: "We suggest the old business adage 'trust but verify.' Ask very specific questions about their references and minute details about the family or work completed. When you check the references, don't tell the reference the information that you were told. Instead ask them open ended questions about the specifics that you were told. For example: Ask 'How do you know (Caregiver's name)?' instead of telling them that you are checking (Caregiver's name) references from when she cared for your dad." In his experience, many applicants give references that are actually personal friends or family and not former supervisors or employers. When this happens, they are eliminated as a candidate.

TRADITIONAL CARE AGENCIES AND ONLINE-BASED CARE COMPANIES

On the surface, it appears that there are more choices than ever to help hire a good professional caregiver for seniors. Thousands of brick and mortar home care agencies are vying for consumers to choose their business. They have beautiful brochures and advertisements in magazines and newspapers and online presences. The Internet-based companies that offer connecting the family directly with caregivers are expanding and massaging the message to consumers to project a more convenient, "so easy" experience to time-hungry customers. Is hiring a good caregiver really evolving to be so breezy that you are just a couple of clicks away from resolving this untidy issue? Not quite yet.

It's true that we are at a crossroads in the home care industry and that many significant factors are at play. Many established companies initially flourished as home health agencies that expanded into the private home care sector. There has been an explosion of companies both big and small in this business. Over time, this industry has become besieged by the ongoing challenges of a shrinking pool of good employees and high employee turnover rates related to the terrible hours, horrible pay, and lack of benefits. There are new federal overtime laws (that may or may not be modified) that require companies to pay overtime as they would in any other employment sector. The traditional agencies are slowly beginning to respond to the pressure to change their pay scales. This has been a shock to the profit margin of traditional home care companies who insist that they should be able to continue to marginalize caregivers as a different class of employees. Many smaller companies are pushed out of business in the competition with major national franchises that take over their local market.

The relatively new kids on the block are the Internet and online-based care companies. The Internet offers convenient options for people wanting to hire privately or with an agency. Not only can you peruse the list of home care agencies in your or your family member's location from anywhere, you can also potentially find reviews for the services of those agencies. From your computer, any search engine can find increasingly diverse hired home care models: websites for traditional home care agencies, employer-caregiver matching websites, and even employment agency–like companies that, for a fee, do the screening and vetting of caregivers for you before you hire privately. This hasn't quite reached the simplicity or reliability of an Amazon product review. However, SeniorAdvisor.com is a good starting point to review competing agencies for some locales, but not all are listed. Yelp can sometimes reveal opinions about a specific agency. The old tried and true method is to ask trusted geriatric care professionals, such as a home health nurse, doctor, hospital discharge planner, or geriatric care manager.

Referred to as online senior care marketplaces or startups, companies such as Care.com, Carelinx.com, Honor.com, and Hometeam.com bring all of the advantages of technology to the hired home care experience. These online senior care websites allow the client to see options for care online and choose caregivers directly with varying levels of assistance in the process. For online-based companies, the market has been well researched and there is much tweaking of the selections and services to meet the demands of elders aging at home and their adult children. (See tables 3.2 and 3.3.) There is essentially no middle man, reducing the cost to the consumer. Reviews and ratings on some sites can be found on the caregiver's information page, making it much simpler for the consumer to weigh pros and cons in their choices.

One of the most innovative trends with the online senior care marketplace and a true departure from the legacy agency model is the evolution of the role of the caregiver. In the legacy tradition, the caregiver is hired by the agency at a low hourly salary and the customer is charged a higher hourly rate. Benefits are rare for those employed by the traditional brick and mortar care agencies and some professional caregivers themselves need government assistance with health care such as Medicaid to survive.

Care.com started the changes with devising a system in which caregivers are free agents, in charge of their own schedules and allowed to negotiate their own higher salaries. But this did not guarantee that they would have payroll taxes processed (though Care.com recommends that to prospective employers) and benefits are not discussed.

The even newer models of online senior care marketplace businesses (such as Honor.com and Carelinx.com) are creating a hybrid of some of the features of a brick and mortar care agency with the convenient features of the Internet and are further remaking the position of the caregiver. Most of these models are establishing their businesses in California and selected U.S. cities. They are slowly in the process of expanding to other states. In this business prototype, the professional caregiver is an employee of the company rather than a person independently contracting their services. The caregiver is a member of the professional team who earns a decent hourly wage, has some benefits, and may even be a shareholder in the company.

This tremendous shift in how the employer treats the caregiver employee is not only laudatory in humanizing this profession, it is also a calculated approach to finding and retaining the best professional caregivers in a fast growing market with a shortage of quality service providers. These companies are betting on being able to entice and retain the very

Table 3.3.   Online Senior Marketplace Companies According to Their Websites

What Online Agency Does and Doesn't Do	Care.com	Honor.com	Carelinx.com
Employer of the caregiver	No	Yes	Yes
Available nationwide	Yes	California, Dallas-Fort Worth, and Albuquerque	California and select cities across the United States
Handles background checks, payroll, taxes, and insurance	Yes and No: Care.com offers HomePay for an additional fee: "provided by Breedlove, takes the work out of paying for care—we do everything from figuring out tax withholdings, setting up payroll or direct deposit, tracking your quarterly taxes and even filing them for you automatically." Offers a convenient background check service	Yes	Yes
Provides training to caregivers for critical knowledge and skills for the job	No	Yes	Not mentioned on their website
Provides initial assessment of the client by a supervisor	No	Yes: "On the first visit, we assess your individual care needs and help design your Care Plan."	Yes: An online survey is assessed by a team member to advise you. Website does not specify what that person's training or background is
Access to caregiver profiles for consumer to choose best fit for the family member	Yes: created and listed by the caregivers themselves	Yes	Yes

Provides expert advice to the consumer throughout the process	Yes: Offers instant chat with a Master's-level geriatric professional	Yes: Honor specialist, usually a Licensed Vocational Nurse. "We're on call 24/7 to make sure you always get the best possible service and support—day or night."	No: However, a team member will assist at the beginning of the hiring process. A phone number is provided for help, but does not specify on website what the help entails or if available 24/7

best of the caregivers out there. They will likely avoid the high employee turnover rate commonly seen in nursing homes and many home care agencies with these same professionals who are largely treated as "the help" and not much better.

There is some evidence that the evolution of fair work practices in the online senior marketplace is having an impact on some brick and mortar care agencies. We have found that some traditional care agencies are raising pay, providing stable hours, and in some cases providing benefits to their employees. Currently, we are mostly seeing this with smaller local or regional companies. It may be that the smaller companies are more nimble and have greater flexibility to make big changes to company policy. They may be able to assess movements and trends in the larger market more quickly. The bigger national franchise companies appear more set in stone. The industry is evolving before our eyes.

It remains to be seen how this will all pan out nationally. But early signs are very promising. It is clear that a better trained, more securely vetted, consumer-rated, and more stable caregiver workforce will be beneficial to the elder receiving care.

INTERVIEW WITH THE CEO OF HONOR.COM SETH STERNBERG

Honor has accomplished setting a new course for consumers of home care services. After entering this market, what adjustments has Honor had to make so far? What were some things that you did not expect and how has the company responded?

A foundational principle at Honor is that care professionals must be well cared for in order to be able to care for others. Through the course of operating a contractor model, we realized there were large limitations to that goal when it came to improving the lives of caregivers. When Honor Care Pros were not employees, we could not train them as we would have liked. We were unable to provide sick time and other benefits that better enable this community to care for their own families. So Honor decided to transition contractors to employees and today we bring all Care Pros onto our platform as employee team members. Any fundamental business model change is challenging; however, one of the strengths of being a more efficient operation is that we can (and want to) experiment with what makes our mission more achievable. Honor came into the industry with open ears and an open mind—we were prepared to adapt quickly to learning in the market.

It's important to note that offering Honor Care Pros training and benefits is important but so is increasing their pay. The national average wage for home care workers is $9.70 an hour. Honor aims to pay more to ensure that our employees can care for themselves and their families. It is not only the right thing to do, it's the best way to make sure Care Pros are able to provide amazing care to our clients.

Another key realization is that technology is the backbone and not the face of the company. It is the human being who walks through the door that customers identify as Honor and the mission is to change the way our loved ones age at home. Honor is powered by people and enhanced by tech. Companies that claim their technology fixes everything are not acknowledging the fact that consumers are not looking for home care because they happen to find an innovative app. They want someone special to come into their lives and care for themselves, a spouse, or parent.

Though technology is not the face of the company, without it Honor would not be able to offer such high-quality care. We are able to construct learning algorithms, monitoring features, and a whole host of client features that allow for transparency and peace of mind. Efficiencies in operations and care management afford us the ability to scale, something that eludes the current industry and keeps it in a very fragmented, hyperlocal state. That is a key insight into why home care looks like it does today—it doesn't benefit from scale and innovation.

A major problem for the customers of traditional care agencies are the state regulations restricting what caregivers can and cannot do in the home to help their clients (give meds, change a simple dressing, give insulin injections, etc.). Even though the customer is paying top dollar for a caregiver through an agency, they are often in a position to find (and pay for) additional help to complete these critical daily tasks for an elder. Are the Honor Care Pros limited by these laws or are they more able to decide with the client and family how to manage these aspects of care, as privately hired caregivers (such as those that would be hired through Care.com) are able to do?

Honor Care Pros absolutely have to adhere to state and local regulations. They do NOT make side arrangements with family to provide service that goes beyond those regulations governing "nonmedical" care.

Does Honor provide geriatric care managers for clients?

Clients have access to our Care Team, which includes LVNs (Licensed Vocational Nurses) with expertise in geriatric care. Here's how Honor works—a client or family member calls or signs up for Honor through the website. Our Care Team assigns a care coordinator to go out to the client's home to note the surroundings, interview the family or care manager in the home, and assess the client's specific needs—that is, mobility, condition-specific care, etc. That profile information goes into our tech platform and through a proprietary algorithm matches that client with the Care Pro in the area with qualifications that match the client's needs. The Care Pro can accept the job through the Care Pro App and receive instructions, a personalized care plan for the client, directions, wellness checklist, client photo and preferences, etc. The Care Pro uses their app to check in and check out as well as leave notes for any other Care Pros who may also be caring for the same client. The client or care manager in the family can rate and give feedback about their visits through the Honor Family App. They can schedule more care, leave notes, and pay for the visit with just a few clicks.

Honor also works closely with health system care managers—for example, if a social worker is looking after the well-being of a senior and we are their home care provider, we communicate with that advocate. We work as a team. In post-acute situations, our Care Pro notes can be shared with designated family and even a client's doctor.

We have made sure that we are tapping the best and brightest minds in health care to ensure that our service is playing a meaningful role in helping people. That's why we have advisors like Dr. Bruce Leff. He is the director of the Center for Transformative Geriatric Research and serves as a professor of Medicine and practicing geriatrician at the Johns Hopkins University School of Medicine. He's the also founder of the Hospital at Home program. Carol Rafael served for twenty-two years as president and CEO of the Visiting Nurse Service of New York and is a nationally recognized expert in health policy and practice. She's chair of the AARP Board and Long Term Quality Alliance. Dr. Ronald Greeno, MD, is the president elect of the Society of Hospital Medicine. He is also the chief strategy officer for IPC Healthcare, Inc. and was the co-founder of Cogent Healthcare Inc., where he developed Cogent's national network of hospitalist physicians.

What is the ongoing supervision for Care Pros like? Do supervisors ever visit the home after the Care Pro has been chosen?

This is a great question. There are a few ways that Care Pros are evaluated and set up for success. First let's look at the Honor technology platform. After the Care Pro checks out of a visit, the family care manager or client receives notes from the visit and the ability to rate the Care Pro as well as give feedback about the visit. Honor's

Care Team follows up with clients to get more detailed information on what can be improved. In addition, technology can continually monitor activity so that alerts are triggered if potentially fraudulent actions occur. For example, GPS tracking can confirm whether a Care Pro arrived at a client's home and verify how long they stayed. This technology also works to protect the Care Pro. If a client claims a Care Pro didn't show up, we can use the data to verify or disprove claims. We have many ways to ensure that Care Pros are providing amazing service . . . and also to make sure Care Pros are safe and set up to succeed at their jobs. Care Pros have twenty-four-hour access to call for help from the Care Team. Through their Care Pro App they can call in sick so the technology and team can find a backup Care Pro for their client.

Is Honor expanding to other states besides California and how will you deal with the different state regulations that deem what a caregiver can and cannot provide in a home setting?

Honor is in the San Francisco Bay area, Los Angeles, and the Dallas-Fort Worth markets. [As of publication, Honor is also in Albuquerque, New Mexico.] We carefully hired general managers with close ties to the local home care and medical communities—who are familiar with local regulations in addition to differences that rest from community to community. Hiring and training is face to face and company culture and processes will be brought into each new location to make sure we are consistent with hiring the best Care Pros who can fill our mission to provide amazing care. Sixty-two million dollars in total funding so far will enable us to grow faster in new cities. We are focused on hiring all the highest quality Care Pros we can get, as well as engineers and local field teams.

As a family member living far away, I love the Honor setup that I could read the caregiver's individual shift reports from anywhere and communicate directly with the caregivers about details of the care that need to be addressed. Many care agencies do not allow this direct communication and require going through the agency as a third party only. How is this aspect of Honor's care going and have there been any problems or concerns?

Families love the reports that we send to those designated to receive them. We have a family who shares responsibility of caring for their dad. Mom handles most of the care. The two grown daughters have children and corporate jobs so they look at care as a team effort with Honor being part of their team. The updates they receive after Care Pro Elaine leaves the home allows all family members to be on the same page. The notes may say, "Dad is having trouble swallowing the new pills, please talk to his doctor. He likes the new cereal, please make sure you pick up more on your way home from work. Dad took a very short nap and may feel tired when Mom gets home, etc." The family has the ability to share the Care Pro updates with doctors or others involved in his care. And what's really valuable to this family in particular is knowing that the Care Pro who is coming later sees all of these notes and can pick up immediately where others left off. There are no notes scribbled on a paper notebook on the table. If there are any issues where a family has questions or concerns, they can flag the Care Team through the app or by phone and that feedback will be kept between them and the Care Team. And any feedback that will help a Care Pro improve in their performance will be shared by the Care Team. Honor is an advocate for both the client and the Care Pro.

How is Honor able to help elders with more advanced needs to remain living at home? For example, keeping people with any type of dementia in their own homes is a huge challenge for families and caregivers. Are there specially trained Care Pros to help people with dementia, immobility and transfers, feeding tubes?

We have Care Pros with specialized training and experience in caring for dementia patients on our platform in addition to those with skills in caring for those with cancer and Parkinson's disease. A

Care Pro's skills with mobility or transfers are all part of their profile so that the matching algorithms won't match a three-hundred-pound patient with cats in the home with a petite Care Pro who is allergic to cats. Because we have partnerships with the American Cancer Society and National Parkinson Foundation—we also have care guidance accessible through the Care Pro App.

In your view, is there an ideal caregiver? If so, what are their characteristics or skills? Are their certain elderly clients who are not appropriate for Honor care? Do you have limits on advanced medical conditions or situations of home care?

One huge insight into the caregiving industry is that both clients and caregivers are all very diverse in their needs, skills, and personalities. The populations are both very heterogeneous, thus you need tools and systems to provide the best match for everyone. What remains the same, however, is that high-quality Care Pros all share one characteristic—they feel deeply satisfied by the act of caring for another person. One woman cared for her grandmother and her family encouraged her to change careers because she was so good at it. Another woman didn't like how her father was treated when he became ill so she decided to get her LVN degree and loves hearing stories from her clients because they remind her of her dad. The skills they all share are patience, compassion, and a sincere respect for older people. Since Honor has such rigid screening and in-person interviews we currently only accept about 5 percent of applicants. These are the people who have that special sparkle in their eye and light up when they see a client. The question we ask when we hire is, "Would I want this person caring for my mom?"

From my own experience hiring caregivers privately for my parents, I know that finding the right people for the job can be like feast or famine. Sometimes it seems that there are simply very few qualified and caring candidates available. How does Honor deal with the fluctuations in the applicant pool?

We find that there's a 65 percent churn rate in the industry because caregivers are also trying to find the right fit. They want to be respected, paid well, and treated like "skilled" professionals. Why does the industry call them "unskilled"? Giving them the ability to see their jobs as careers and balance their own lives while becoming better at what they do is the key. Honor has seen the churn rate dip to as low as 15 percent with many of our Care Pro men and women moving into careers as RNs. We need to transform the way customers, healthcare systems, and the general public see home caregivers. Caregiving is one of the fastest growing jobs in the world due to the ever-increasing need for professional care. They are vital to our health system and very important to families.

INTERVIEW WITH A "CARE PRO" FROM HONOR.COM

What was your interest in becoming a professional caregiver?

I take care of my own family. It gives me a sense of fulfillment to take care of people whether they are my own children or older people. I'm at peace when I know somebody is having a better life. I like meeting new people and when they trust you to take care of their family member, it's very rewarding. I feel important. I have families from years back that still call me, even after their loved one has passed.

What has your work experience been like before working for Honor? Did you work in a nursing or assisted living facility? Home care agency?

Before Honor, I worked for sixteen years at different places, including an assisted living facility and for placement agencies. I've seen it all. With the agencies I would be told to go to someone's house without knowing much about the client. Sometimes the client would want to hire me just to work with their family and not go through an agency.

What are the best and worst parts of your job?

The trust that a family has in you feels amazing. And I know that I am making someone's life or situation better. I like knowing that I am helping a client and sometimes relieving a family member who is caring for a loved one and just needs help. The worst part of being a caregiver, before Honor, was not knowing how to advance in my career. I don't have a nursing degree, so I always felt that I could never move up, no matter how well I do my job. But at Honor I know that I am an important employee. I will be able to receive training and get even better at my job. I feel there's hope.

How long have you worked for Honor?

I've worked for Honor since November 2015. They respect my expertise and appreciate the service that I give. I can manage my time, life, work. For the first time, I have a choice in the jobs that I accept. And I feel respected and connected to the company and to other Care Pros.

How is working for Honor different for you than your previous caregiver jobs?

For sixteen years I've been doing this job and this is the first time I've had something like this Care Pro App on my phone. With other agencies, you call them and they give you what jobs they have and you have to take it or leave it. And with the Care Pro App technology I can receive and accept a care request through my phone. Information about the client comes from an Honor assessor who has met with the client face to face. That information goes into the app. Information about me, my skills, my location, and experience are also in the app. So the technology makes the best matches between clients and Care Pros. I have a chance to accept or decline a job request. I can read notes about the client before I go to the house, so I know what to expect. After I'm finished interacting with the client, I can also make sure that the next Care Pro has notes from me so he or she can pick up where I left off. So the patient is always getting the best care. The family can also see our notes so they are in the loop and they can rate our performance so we always have feedback. You always know how you're doing because you get "stars" on the app.

What is your advice to families who are looking to hire a caregiver?

I can't tell families what to do, but I have seen everything and I can see that it's very important that the client is comfortable. If your family member really wants to stay at home there are experienced, caring people who really want to help. You should make sure you are very clear with what you need and how you want your loved one to be cared for. What are your preferences? Ask "What makes him or her most comfortable?" The caregiver should be physically able to perform the job. For example, is he or she able to lift the client if needed? And find a company that gives strict background checks. I've had them before, but the one Honor did before I was hired was the most thorough I've ever had.

TAKEAWAY POINTS FOR THIS CHAPTER

- Look at the requirements to become a Certified Nursing Assistant in your state. Ask the agency you are considering hiring what certification their employees have, what training they offer beyond those state requirements, and how often they offer training.
- Find your state's regulations regarding tasks that personal care aides and Certified Nursing Assistants can do in the home. If hiring with an agency, ask if this will impact your family member's particular situation.
- Once you have a clear picture of the gaps (special medication, dressing changes, etc.) in the coverage you need to arrange for, you can make decisions about how to fill those daily needs. Supplement with family help, privately hired care for specific tasks, home health coverage, or possibly other state-sponsored care programs.
- When ready to hire, take a look at some options available in your area and choose one. Remember, if you don't like how it works out, you can always try a different one or a combination of services.
- If you are hiring privately, *always* do a thorough background check and verification of who the applicant is.
- Take a look at the hybrid online senior care businesses if they are available in your area. They do offer convenience with finding caregivers and not having to worry about payroll and taxes and usually have a

transparent, lower price. They may vary in the level of ongoing support that you may have with a brick and mortar care agency.

- Most importantly, realize that to meet the needs of your family, you may hire through a home care agency, hire privately, or any combination of both. There is no one right way, only the way that works for your elder and their situation.

4

BUILDING THE BEST CARE PARTNERSHIP

The hope of every family seeking a caregiver is to find "the one" that is a good fit. So many factors are involved when choosing a caregiver and some of these are not under your control. Building the best care partnership takes planning, commitment, and an attitude of flexibility. The elder may not be on board with the idea, your agency doesn't have the available staff for you to pick and choose, scheduling requires multiple caregivers, and family members disagree about who is needed and how much care is needed. Do the best you can do and let the chips fall where they may! Unintended consequences are inevitable. But fear not, we will guide you through the process of finding and keeping "the one."

Everyone who is involved with helping a family member stay in their home needs a bit of encouragement now and then. You may think that you do not have the skills to handle making the arrangements to hire good caregivers in your or your parents' home. You may have moments that you think you are not cut out for this. You are not alone. Very few people come fully equipped to deal with all aspects of this care. Taking a step back to assess your own readiness for this venture is a good idea. As the family "manager," here are the main skills and qualities that you need at the outset to make a caregiving arrangement go smoothly:

- Patience with people. You will need patience with the hiring process, with the newly hired caregiver, with the elder's adjustment to having a person helping them, and with problems that naturally arise.

- Willingness to give your time when necessary. Time is precious; you must be willing to give the time needed for your parent's care arrangement. Can you carve out time to regularly check in on your parent and the caregiver and to read caregiver notes to make sure tasks are being completed? This can mean unexpected interruptions of work and family time that require your immediate attention when issues come up.
- Motivation to make it work. If you are not really committed to the idea that staying at home rather than moving to an assisted living is the best option, it probably isn't going to work.
- Ability to delegate whenever possible. This is a job that can be a very long haul. If you are inclined to hesitate to hand over part of the job to another because of guilt, embarrassment, or need to control everything, get over it! Whether you are the spouse, the adult children, or the person needing care, be mindful of enlisting others to do tasks when and where you can.
- Willingness to accept that the arrangement will not always be perfect and that you can't control every aspect of the care. Flexibility, compromise, and acceptance will become your mantra.
- Know where you have support for your role and your own self-care. Do you have a spouse or partner who can listen to you recount your efforts with patience? Do you have friends who are in the same boat and managing their own parents' care either at home or in an assisted living situation? Having real people who can help you process out loud and problem solve with you is priceless during this operation. Becoming isolated is very problematic for family caregivers and family managers. For some, this can lead to anxiety and depression. Do you have someone that you can be your "second in command" when you go on a business trip or fly to your best friend's daughter's wedding? In some families, care of the parents tends to fall on one sibling. But if another sister or brother is willing to hold down the fort intermittently, that is valuable to the sanity and peace of mind of the one in charge.

As you read this, you are most likely considering hiring a caregiver to assist with a parent or other family member. Coming to this conclusion can be fraught with anguish and anxiety. Your situation may be one characterized by an elder's slow decline or the result of an illness or accident, recent hospitalization, memory problems, or any number of other situations that call for help in the home. Typically family members are more overwrought than the elder themselves! We all feel a responsibility and an urgent need to *do something* immediately.

Take a deep breath. Unless it is a real emergency, you should take the time to think things through and do your best to make this a positive and sustainable option. The previous chapters have provided a road map to choosing an agency or other source of caregivers and determining training requirements. We discussed ways to broach the subject of care in chapter 2 and will expand upon that topic here. In your haste to solve the problem you may make the grave mistake of neglecting to get your elder on board with the idea. Even after persuading an elder to go along with initiating home care, resistance can occur at any stage of the process, especially at the beginning. By resistance we mean an ongoing opposition or outright refusal to accept care. This can be in the form of verbal complaints, avoidance, anger, passivity, or change in mood or disposition. As irritating and complicating as this may be to you, it can be emotionally draining for an elder to maintain this resistance. For an elder with dementia, bringing a stranger into the home can cause fear, confusion, and anger, all of which can increase agitation. Pay attention to what you see, hear, and observe and offer support and reassurance. Examine the situation closely to determine if perhaps the caregiver is not a good fit or the caregiver approach needs tweaking. As people get older, independence becomes a huge issue. None of us wants to admit we need help with the tasks that define us as competent individuals. Work, family life, social engagement, driving, finances, and all the other tasks and goals that we take for granted become severely compromised. Even for elders who recognize there may be some creeping problems with everyday tasks, they may not want to burden their children or have too much pride to admit they can't manage like before. Be kind, considerate, and respectful.

Resistance and frustration can occur at any time throughout the process. And these emotions don't just come from the elder. Family members can disagree about whether help is even needed or how much help should be considered. What about costs? Will the family share in costs? Who will take the lead in making decisions about care and who will talk to mom or dad about bringing care into the home? A family meeting, even by phone, can help to clarify some of these questions. Typically a particular family member has been "the responsible one." If that person is you, make certain you bring other family members into the discussion to avoid problems later on. As you read this book, you may be much better prepared to tackle the idea of home care than your siblings or another parent. Educate and inform family members on what you know. Be patient and discuss how the costs of care will be handled by the family so that these issues are definitively settled.

We have seen numerous situations in which one adult child lives near mom or dad and has taken on most of the responsibility of care. Resentment, entitlement, and expectations can affect the discussion. Proximally distant family members may become overly involved or not involved enough. Be patient and do your best to reach consensus.

If your family situation is so untenable that decisions can't be made, consider an elder care mediator to help sort through disagreements. In most cases, family members can reach agreement about how to approach the situation with one person being designated as the "spokesperson" to talk to the elder. Remember that family members can have some of the same reactions to the idea of care as the elder.

Most of us have difficulty accepting that a parent is getting older and needs help. After all, our parents have taken care of us our whole lives and this gradual role reversal can be emotionally challenging. Family members can have dramatically different views of how mom and dad are doing. A sister may state: "Mom and dad are doing fine! They are just getting a bit older and slower." A brother may have the complete opposite reaction and want to ship mom and dad to an assisted living facility as soon as possible! Conflicting feelings, agendas, and motivations all influence how family members react to a change in an elder's situation.

HIRING CAREGIVERS BECOMES A FAMILY AFFAIR

Thomas and Kate's Story

Joseph is a ninety-seven-year-old man who now has twenty-four-hour caregiving. His son, Thomas, and Thomas's wife, Kate, live nearby. The trajectory of their story is not unlike thousands of other stories that tell of the frustrations and trials and errors of finding caregivers for family members.

It all started when Joseph's wife, Barbara, was still alive. Her health had begun to deteriorate and Joseph was recuperating from knee replacement surgery. Kate began to spend many hours a week tending to their needs: grocery shopping, going for medications, cooking meals, and doing laundry. It got to the point where Kate could no longer manage all the care required. A local agency was contacted and they provided a caregiver for a few hours a day to assist with these tasks. Then Barbara died suddenly. Joseph was left alone without his wife of many years. Thomas and Kate decided to continue providing the already established caregiving to Joseph. The caregiver took him out to eat, provided transportation to appointments, and helped with showers, cooking, and cleaning. And then Joseph's health began to worsen. He fell several times during the night and had to go the ER after these falls, necessitating that Kate and Thomas had to come over in the middle of the night. It became exhausting. And clearly Joseph's safety was at risk.

Thomas and Kate decided that Joseph needed twenty-four-hour care. They contacted the agency for additional caregivers to augment the hours currently being provided. As Thomas states, "Using an agency turned out to be more expensive and the quality of the caregivers was disappointing. People were sent over that varied wildly from those that were wonderful to those that should not be alone in the house with my father. We decided to strike out on our own and hire people privately. We received some recommendations from a friend who is a nurse and were able to piece together twenty-four-hour care with revolving shifts. Although there have been crises, hassles, and challenges with managing the caregivers, it has proved to be far better than going with an agency."

Joseph's Story

Joseph, although very old, still retains his intellectual capacity. This is a man who knows what he wants and is not afraid to ask for it. In that way he is similar to many older people, but he is unlike many others who have memory problems associated with dementia or other medical problems. Joseph's story mostly mirrors Thomas's with the exception that Joseph does not feel he needs twenty-four-hour care, although he accepts it. He still views himself as capable of doing more things than he really can. Joseph is mostly confined to a wheelchair, although he can walk short distances with a walker. He needs help with showers, toileting, shopping, cooking, and cleaning. Most of all, however, Joseph enjoys getting out of the house. His caregivers take him to the park to watch people and enjoy the fresh air and he goes out to eat and to the symphony and states that these excursions are what he requires of any caregiver that works for him.

Joseph has strong views on the caregiving industry. He went through numerous caregivers from agencies that he says "were incompetent, dishonest, and didn't care." Joseph confirms that he, Thomas, and Kate decided to hire someone not through an agency. They took recommendations from friends and colleagues. The process was not seamless. There were the inevitable crises and challenges, but everyone agrees that it was worth it. Joseph is very clear about what he thinks are the important qualities of a caregiver:

- Being observant: A caregiver must anticipate what the elder needs and wants by paying close attention to body language and emotion.
- Memory: A caregiver needs to remember the process of how a task was done and do it the same way each time. Joseph uses the example of taking a shower. Assisting someone with this intimate task takes multiple steps that should be performed the same way each time, paying attention to the details.
- Caring: Joseph says that it is obvious when someone doesn't care or doesn't want to be there.

Joseph has some strong opinions about the future of the caregiving industry. In addition to the reasons mentioned, the federal overtime requirement instituted on January 1, 2016, which mandates that caregivers be paid time and a half if they work over eight hours a day, has made hiring caregivers from an agency "unaffordable for most people." Joseph believes that caregivers will "leave agencies in droves to be hired privately." The advantages he sees are that the caregivers make more and the consumer pays less. Joseph states that even though his caregivers have other jobs as well, they prefer to work for him privately rather than through an agency. When asked about whether he had any kind of liability insurance to protect himself, he said he didn't feel that was necessary in his case and that he has his caregivers "sign something" that states they will pay their own taxes.

Joseph is very happy with his current caregiving situation and when asked about what he would do in the event that one or more of his aides left his employment, he said he would ask for referrals from people he trusted in the community.

Joseph's situation isn't unique, but it is also not necessarily typical of many other families faced with hiring caregivers. Joseph is competent, meaning he is an active participant in the decision-making process.

TACTICS FOR DEALING WITH RESISTANCE AND REJECTION

You need to anticipate resistance or outright rejection, that way you won't be so shocked and defensive when it occurs. Being forewarned is being forearmed. Take a moment to think about why your elder might not want some stranger coming to their home. Consider the following possibilities of why your elder has strong emotional reactions to the idea of bringing a stranger into their home and what might be going on in their mind:

- "I haven't had a chance to clean the house! I can't possibly have some stranger come in to see me."
- "I am a perfectly independent person who has managed for this many years. I don't need someone to take care of me. I am not a baby."
- "I may be having a little trouble here and there, but certainly nothing that I can't manage on my own."
- "This is an expense that is unnecessary and that I simply can't afford."

A stranger coming into the home can be viewed as being intrusive, disruptive, invasive, and threatening. Acknowledge and truly try and understand these emotions before approaching the idea of a caregiver. Remember: show empathy and respect during the discussion.

We have used a few examples in chapter 2 on how to approach an elder with the idea of hiring a caregiver by planning ahead using tact and an incremental approach. If your elder has dementia, a somewhat different approach will be needed, but here are some suggestions on how to approach someone who has the capacity to make their own decisions:

- Approach the conversation from a stance of partnership. We are in this together and will make decisions together. I am not here to tell you what to do.
- Provide a basic and truthful explanation of the problems you observe.
- Agree to disagree. Listen and accept what the other person has to say. Fighting about any differences of opinion will not help.
- If the conversation is not going well, defer to a different day.
- Make the suggestion of "trying" a caregiver out for a defined period of time, at which point you both revisit the situation and make changes accordingly. But if you are going to do this, mean it and stick to it.

Before we talk about the difficult and challenging task of helping someone who has dementia, consider Sam's story.

Sam is a robust, affable man who is ninety-five years old. He was a star basketball player in his youth and he retains the lanky physique of an athlete. Sam has also been diagnosed with Alzheimer's disease. Most days he is happy and grateful, but on other days he is confused, repeats the same stories over and over again, and obsesses about money. Although Sam has managed pretty well in his own home, he has left the front door unlocked and given personal information over the phone to scammers. His hygiene has been poor—his clothes are disheveled and he clearly has not taken a shower as often as he should. His family questions whether he is getting enough to eat because food sits in his fridge and he is losing weight. Sam's wife died many years ago so he is all alone and doesn't drive any longer.

Sam has expressed a strong desire to stay in his home with his beloved dog, Pepper. His family decides it is time to consider hiring caregivers to come to Sam's home during the day to help him with meals, laundry, showering, and getting him out in the community so he can be around other people.

When the family suggests this idea to Sam, he is incensed. In his booming voice he proclaims, "I don't need anyone to take care of me. Things are going just fine!" The family persists in their efforts to try and convince him to allow someone in and Sam throws up the same wall of resistance.

The family decides to try something both bold and risky. They decide to simply bring a caregiver over to the home, introduce her to Sam, and see how things go. The first day this occurs, Sam is gracious and polite. As time goes on, Sam complains from time to time about "help I don't need," but several months later he has come to completely accept the presence of the care staff. In fact, he verbalizes how wonderful they are and how much companionship they provide. Sam has gained weight, he goes to the senior center and out shopping with the aide, and they walk his dog Pepper so he gets some much needed exercise. As Sam's symptoms of dementia have worsened, the hours that caregivers come in have been increased and eventually he may need overnight care.

A word of caution: It doesn't always go like this. We have seen situations in which elders are so angry and upset by the idea of someone coming into the home that there appears to be no viable solution to the problem of desperately needed help in the home. If you are uncertain about whether your elder has dementia, begin with a complete medical workup followed by an evaluation for dementia by a trained geriatric professional. If you haven't already, educate yourself about the symptoms and behaviors associated with dementia. A good place to start is the Alzheimer's Association.[1] The obstinate and unreasonable behavior sometimes exhibited by a person with dementia can be extremely frustrating. Patience is required. Arguing will only exacerbate the situation. Expect to repeat whatever plan you have made as often as needed and with patience and resolve. Gently remind the elder that this was a plan that was agreed to at an earlier time and we are now proceeding.

CHOOSING THE BEST AGENCY

If you live in a community that has many private duty agencies to choose from, the following are some suggestions on how to find a good agency. Keep in mind that many states do not require licensure of any kind to open a home care agency.[2]

- Ask friends and colleagues if they have had experiences with an agency. You may be surprised at how many people have hired caregivers when you ask.

- Talk to your local outreach program with the Area Agency on Aging. Their staff often have experience with agencies and their ombudsman program may have had complaints on certain agencies.
- Call a geriatric care manager and ask his or her opinion.
- Consult with a geriatric physician's office and ask for a list of references.
- Check your local Better Business Bureau and see if there are complaints about an agency you are considering.

Communication with an agency is critical. You are not their only customer, but they should treat you as if you are. Questions to ask include:

- Who do I call in case of emergency or if there is a problem?
- Who is responsible for scheduling changes?
- What is the protocol for missed visits?
- Does the agency do background checks and drug screening?
- Can I communicate directly with the caregivers or do I have to go through the agency?
- Is there someone to reach twenty-four hours a day?
- Ask to review the contract for services.

Personal care agencies continue to try and set themselves apart in new and unique ways. Try and find an agency that resonates with your needs and philosophy of care.

INTERVIEW WITH MELISSA ANDERSON, CO-OWNER OF HOME CARE ASSISTANCE

Author's Note: Home Care Assistance is a senior care franchise. In 2012 there were thirty-five different senior care franchise companies in the United States.[3] Home Care Assistance, like other franchised companies, has locations throughout the country. Because each location is typically separately owned and operated, there may be significant variability in the quality and management of each company.

Why did you get into this business?

As a family we took care of our grandma and we didn't know there were options, programs, and resources to help us take care of her other than facility care. We are passionate about allowing seniors to age in place where they are most comfortable. It was a business that just made sense for us. My dad and I are co-owners of Home Care Assistance. He does marketing and hiring and I run the day-to-day operations. Of all the home care franchises available we chose Home Care Assistance, because it was started by geriatric psychologists and their corporate offices provide senior care services. We also believe Home Care Assistance is really on the cutting edge of research and appreciate the proprietary programs they have implemented.

What sets you apart from other agencies?

We have programs that are unique to us. Home Care Assistance has what we call the Balance Care Method. We train our caregivers not just to do ADLs (Activities of Daily Living), but how to know and work with the whole person. We approach care from an emotional, physical, and spiritual place. There is an emphasis on calmness and purpose, social ties, balanced diet, physical activity, etc. We train our staff to focus on increasing quality of life and addressing these areas of the Balanced Care Method. It is like Maslow's hierarchy of needs. Address basic needs but build on things from there. At HCA we want to change lives for the better. When we are able to make a nice meal and invite friends over because a senior can't host that party anymore and provide that stimulation that is very important. Initially we meet with the family and try and get a sense of what they used to do and they aren't doing any more. Could mobility be an issue and is home health needed? Or is there a physical therapy routine already in place that we can assist with? We use a Balance Care sheet—what are the activities that our clients enjoy and how can we assist with helping clients access those important elements? Our clients need to be valued and our care staff is privileged to work with them. Our staff is not there to just to sit and provide simple companionship. There is so much more that is important.

Home Care Assistance also has a program called Cognitive Therapeutics. Many companies train their caregivers to work with behaviors that may arise with someone who is suffering from memory loss, which is so important. We do that too. In addition, we train our caregivers to work with clients to stimulate them mentally. The program was designed by a neuropsychologist. It works on memory, language, visual spatial relations, executive functioning, coping, etc. We believe that this approach helps with behaviors by providing a sense of purpose and keeping people busy and active. We have seen this program help our clients to have less agitation and frustration. We have an interventionist who does one-on-one cognitive training, and we train certain caregivers in this method, as well. We recommend twelve visits with an interventionist and then our trained caregivers take over.

We also have a veteran's assistance program that helps veterans and their spouses look into the Aid and Attendance pension to help pay for the long-term care costs. We have partnered with a company that assists with the paperwork and then determines if they are a good candidate for the pension. If they are, we can start the care before the VA approves the application at no out-of-pocket expense for the veteran/spouse.

What is your biggest challenge and how do you retain staff?

The biggest challenge is finding qualified caregivers. We only hire about one in twenty-five applicants. We want skilled individuals that have experience with ADLs. We find our caregivers mostly from word of mouth from staff we already have and from sites like Indeed and MyCNAJobs.com. We also hire CNAs right out of school and offer to help pay back their tuition costs after they work with us for a certain amount of time. We offer a health plan where we pay our employee's co-pay and they or anyone in their family can talk to a doctor at any time and we pay the monthly fee. We admire and appreciate our caregivers. They have a hard job. We do barbeques; we do a lot of recognition—texts, phone calls. We are proud to say that we have received the Best of Home Care Employer of Choice award for the last three years. We try to give caregivers the hours they need, but it is in constant flux. A lot of caregivers work two part-time jobs at different agencies. Before caregivers could pick one agency and work as much as they wanted. Now they can't do that due to the federal overtime pay requirement. Some of our caregivers work for another agency so they can get their forty hours if that is what they need. Our client contract stipulates that the consumer cannot hire the caregiver privately. We have to protect our assets and there is a fee associated with hiring our caregivers away.

How does your staff communicate with family members?

Communication between care staff and family is typically through the documentation the caregiver provides on the client daily. A care note left in the house in a binder. We may eventually go to electronic charting. We get copies of the documentation and file in our office. The family can have access to the notes any time they want. A care manager does an in-home visit approximately twice a month to assess how things are going. That visit is followed by an update to the family. There is also a family room portal online where families can see schedules and who is coming to the house. We want families to communicate with us if there is a problem with a caregiver. Communication with family members is tailored to each family.

Who are your caregivers?

I have read that 30 percent of home care companies have been impacted by caregiver shortage. Our caregivers are a range of people. We hire CNAs right out of school or are going to nursing school. Some of them are with us for years and the stress is lower than working in an assisted living. Our caregivers are diverse from many different ethnicities and cultures and we love having them on our team. The important quality we look for is someone who has the skills that we need.

CHOOSING THE BEST CAREGIVER

Choosing the best caregiver may mean having no choice at all. If you live out of town or don't have the time to personally interview or even meet a potential candidate, you may have to handle the situation over the phone. In either case, think about the kind of person your elder might relate best with. Quite frankly, this is where things can get a bit tricky. There may be clear preferences that may need to be overlooked due to federal antidiscrimination laws. We have seen numerous situations in which a family member may think they know the kind of person that would be best suited to mom or dad and the complete opposite turns out to be the case. The lesson is: as much as you want to control the situation, you may just have to let the chips fall where they may and see how things go. That being said, here are some examples to consider as absolutes or as a "wish list":

- Male or female? This can be a clear and legitimate consideration. Many females simply don't want a male assisting them. That can be a good thing because there are many more female caregivers and males can be difficult to find.[4]
- Introvert or extrovert? This one can be tough to predict because sometimes a "talker" may actually be better for someone who is typically more withdrawn. The conversation can actually be beneficial for a person who has become isolated from social engagement. On the other hand, an elder can also be in great need of someone who is comfortable to listen to them talk.
- Housekeeper or white glove patrol? Most caregivers are expected to do some light house cleaning with the job. Some are much more interested in cleaning than others. Believe it or not, this issue comes up for many clients as they either want someone who is more fastidious than they are or they don't want someone disturbing loved but dusty collectibles. Even though you may tell your family member that the person is a caregiver, they may still see the caregiver's role as for the purpose of cleaning. One elder on an outing with her caregiver was asked who the caregiver was. With no ill intent, she replied, "She's the cleaning lady, she goes with me everywhere."

BOOST YOUR CAREGIVER CONNECTION: BUILD GOOD COMMUNICATION FROM THE START

When you and your family have finally hired a caregiver, you will hope for that magical moment when your elder family member and the caregiver click. You see that they seem to understand each other; your father who almost never has something nice to say about this arrangement suddenly compliments something the caregiver has done for him; the caregiver seems to know just when to give your mom space and yet has somehow convinced her to take a bath. Yes, it really can and does happen. After all of your effort to set up this arrangement, you can feel the tension ease and you feel a renewed confidence that this is really going to work.

With any caregiving situation, you want to bolster the positive results and consistent care with good, clear communication. You could read many books by many experts about how to communicate effectively. It's likely, however, that you don't really have time for that. What we will discuss here are some essential areas to cover and describe some effective tools for you to use.

Let's start with the priorities.

The Caregiving Tasks: Some caregivers are better than others at coming into a care situation and having the experience or the intuition to see what needs to be done. Never assume that they will automatically know what your family member needs help with. For example, if your mother needs a person standing by while she takes a shower for safety, but would be embarrassed if someone came in and tried to shampoo her hair while she was showering, you must explain that clearly.

Tool: A written list on a log sheet (see the Sample Caregiver Log Sheets later in this chapter) for private hires or a care plan with a care agency is essential to describe what actions must take place, when, and how frequently. For families that only have one caregiver who only comes for part of the day, communication is pretty direct between the elder, the family, and the caregiver. Not too much gets lost. However, if you have more than one caregiver, it is critical for caregivers to communicate and see changes that are happening over a week or a day. A log sheet is a great tool to use for this scenario. One RN home care manager we know tells the home care staff: "Once any new caregiver arrives, you will facilitate a person to person shift change report, using the log sheet as your guide. Once you arrive for your morning shift, review the log sheet from the previous day, and update the other caregiver(s)." The combination of the written log sheet and the person to person communication allows questions to be answered and information to be clarified, such as: "What is the transportation to the doctor's office tomorrow? Who is picking up the prescription? Did the home health nurse visit yesterday? I don't see it on the log sheet." If you live far away, you can request that at the end of the day, the caregiver on duty takes a photo of the completed log sheet and sends it to you by text or e-mail. Another important aspect of a log sheet is that it can be updated as needed. Remember that aging can be a fluid process, with changes back and forth. Keep the log sheet in a format that is easily edited as things change. When working with an agency, it is imperative that you understand their communication system with their staff. Do they write an online narrative note to communicate with their supervisor and other caregivers? Do you as the customer have access to that? What do they do if there is an unexpected event or problem encountered?

Other tools: Isn't there an app for that? We are in the age of helpful applications for smartphones and computers to communicate specific information rapidly.[5] We know some clever family members who have created their own app so that they can have direct communication with caregivers in order to know exactly when a caregiving task has been completed. But do not fear if you are not a tech whiz who can create an app for your mom. There are lots of new apps coming on the scene to help with elder care. One that we like that has lots of potential for elders, caregivers, and family members is CareZone,[6] available on iPhone, Android, and on your laptop. You can use their tracker feature to store blood glucose levels, blood pressure, pain, mood, sleep, and weight, to name a few. The journal on CareZone can be used for observations or noting changes. It also has a calendar to remind everyone of appointments and a handy medication scanner that you can use to take photos of pill bottles (or type in if you prefer) to accurately keep an up-to-date list of medications with refill dates. They even have a pharmacy feature to purchase pills that come in individual time of day packets. All of this and a "Share With" section so that you can control who gets access. You give access to family members and caregivers to get the information that they need and they in return can share with you.

Personal preferences and history: We all hope for a long-term caregiver who gets to know and build a great relationship with our loved one over time. Some caregivers don't work out though, and it is good to be prepared for change. When a new caregiver comes into to the picture or your parent's care needs change and there is an additional caregiver, it can ease the transition if you have a consistent plan for describing your family member's personality and preferences.

Tool: If you are the elder and are fully able to communicate, make sure that you spend the time with the caregiver to share something about who you are and what your personal preferences are. If you are a family member of an elder who is less able to do this for themselves, and you live nearby and have time, you can sit down with your parent and the caregiver to discuss their preferences about food, what they like to wear, how and where they want the kitchen dishes to be put away, what not to touch in their home, etc. If you don't live near your parent, a simple notebook with this type of general information and some chronological photos or written description to describe what your parent has done in their lifetime and some reference to their work, hobbies, and interests can give the caregiver a visual reference to your parent and who they have been over their lifespan. This is especially helpful if your parent has any form of dementia or limited ability to talk, such as with the aftermath of a stroke or Parkinson's disease.

What to do in an emergency or unusual situation: Of course, for medical issues you are going to be prepared and have all the necessary documents ready for an emergency (see Tools just below). But what about other events that may have to do with the home or outside intrusions? There are power outages, clogged toilets, or broken microwaves. Depending on whether your parent's home is independently owned or has a maintenance service built in, this can be confusing for a caregiver to know what to do. More insidious are phone solicitors and strangers who knock on the door. There are a lot of scams aimed at defrauding the elderly. We will discuss security in greater detail in chapter 5. At this point, though, keep in mind that a caregiver may not know how you want them to respond.

Tools: The caregiver needs to know what documents are needed for what situations and where they are. Though doctor's offices are supposed to have current lists of meds and the medical history in their charts and online systems, they often require it from the patient at every visit. A printed recent medical history and medication list are essential for an elder's home. These can be placed in a designated notebook to be taken with the person for every doctor's visit. If your parent no longer carries a wallet or purse, their Medicare and insurance cards and photo ID need to be with the notebook or a reminder to take these vital documents as well.

Copies of the Do Not Resuscitate Orders that are signed by the elder should also be kept safely in this notebook or another reliable spot in the elder's home easily found by the caregiver or EMT staff.

Regarding nonmedical but unusual events, make the basics of home maintenance clear to caregivers. If there is building management such as in a condo or rental home, have the number available and accessible. The same goes for communicating if different family members take responsibility for different maintenance problems. For example, if your sister is the master plumber of the family, but you take care of calls to the utilities, jot that down in the general information section of your notebook. Include all emergency contacts.

For those annoying and potentially financially destructive telemarketers and scam callers, use caller ID to screen out nuisance calls as much as possible. Though there is the government "No Call List," most people do not find it effective. Initiated in 2003, it currently cannot screen out robocalls and excludes political campaign solicitors.[7] This can be difficult, especially for people with dementia. They want to answer their own phone, but can be easily targeted. Remember that the landline phone is a resource with much more significance for the older generation. The landline phone has served as a mainstay for communication and connection to the outside world for decades for people before there were cell phones, computers, e-mails, texting, instant chat, social media, and video calls.[8] We will discuss in chapter 5 how to balance this vital and familiar piece of home equipment and safety.

SAMPLE CAREGIVER LOG SHEETS

This log sheet example is for a person who has fairly simple needs and a caregiver who is with them for only part of the day:

Smith Family Caregiver Log: Alice

Date: _____

1. Meals (note percentage eaten or refused): Breakfast _____ Lunch_____
2. Bathing and dressing: With assist _____ With supervision _____
3. Medications: Morning _____ Evening _____
4. Activities (please note any exercise, walks, visits, shopping, doctor's visits, or other daytime activities): _____

   _____

   _____

This log sheet example is for:

- A person who has twenty-four-hour care
- A person who has any memory problems or difficulty communicating
- Any complex medical issues or medications administered more often than twice a day
- A situation with more than one caregiver, especially agency caregivers who may not have been to this case before

Especially if you are hiring from an agency and do not have access to the agency's notes, having your family's own log sheet can reduce miscommunication.

Walker Family Caregiver Log: Jim

Date: _____

Caregivers and shift: Day _____ Evening _____ Night _____

Meals (note percentage eaten or if refused): Breakfast _____ Lunch_____ Snacks _____ Dinner _____

Bathing and dressing: With assist _____ With supervision _____

Medications: Morning _____ Noon _____ Dinner _____ Bedtime _____

Mood Changes (note good, fair, bad, behavior): _____

Day _____ Evening/Night _____

Pain (note time, where pain is, action taken, and response):

_____

Activities (please note any exercise, walks, visits, outings, doctor's visits, or other day/evening activities): _____

_____

Problems or concerns: _____

Good communication is essential in every aspect of life and the setting of a family with a hired caregiver is no exception. We know a daughter-in-law who is a queen of communication in our view. While she is very clear about what she wants for her family member who is receiving care, she expresses herself with kindness but without being fawning or manipulative. Her communication style exemplifies what we think of as the three keys to successful communication with a care agency or caregiver:

1. Be firm: Say what you want to be done clearly and as concisely as possible. Repeat the message as consistently as possible. Do so as needed with an even, neutral tone and without anger or sarcasm.
2. Be fair: Understand that some of what you want may not be possible or even necessary. Listen to the feedback from the caregiver and make sure that every party is on the same page and comprehends the goal.
3. Be friendly: Most caregivers we know truly want to do what is best for their client. If you are asking for something to be done and it is not, make time to go over it and clarify. While it can be frustrating, it will do more harm than good to express annoyance to or take out your anger on a caregiver who is usually trying to do their best. If they aren't, you simply need a new caregiver. Keep in mind: some agencies don't allow families to directly communicate to the caregiver what they want to be on the care plan, but insist that the family only communicate this to staff at the agency. This is another layer of potential miscommunication and the caregiver can be stuck in the middle if the directive is not clear to them.

Be honest with yourself so that you can be as accountable as you want the caregiver or care agency to be. Have you really clearly explained to a talkative caregiver how much your parent detests any sort of chattering or have you just hinted at it? On the flip side, you may be avoiding dealing directly with your parent about what you view as an unrealistic demand or complaint about a caregiver. Even as an adult, it can be hard to disagree with your parent about some things. The best thing to do is talk it through.

TAKEAWAY POINTS FOR THIS CHAPTER

- Before the hiring process begins, get family members on board and do your best to reach consensus.
- Don't be hard on yourself if you are not an expert on how to put the parts together immediately. It comes with practice and time. Delegate whenever you can.
- Assess and deal with resistance. Be patient during the process.
- If your elder has dementia, educate yourself about this challenging and devastating disease.
- Take your time in finding an agency. Try to get firsthand referrals from reputable sources.
- Use different tools to communicate clear expectations of what needs to be done for your family member and have a system of checking that items are completed.
- Be firm, fair, and friendly in your communication with the caregiver and the care agency. Never use the caregiver as someone to complain to. Have others in your support circle be your sounding board.

5

KEEP YOUR EYE ON THE BALL

Security and legal protections are a top priority for families that choose to hire caregivers, whether you hire them privately or through a trusted care agency. From the beginning, smart families will do due diligence in checking on references and previous jobs, require background checks, drug screening before hiring, and random checks after employment, and an employee contract. The more you can do up front in the process, the better.

Let's have a reality check though. If you have been reading this book, you are making an effort to hire care either for yourself or a loved one. You are trying to do it the very best way possible. Can you do every one of these steps simultaneously and ensure that every aspect of the care is completely perfect and safe? Of course not. And you cannot do it completely alone. We want to take this moment to emphasize that you will delegate tasks out of necessity. When it comes to security, the more help you can get from trusted people, the better. Even with the top of the line security systems in place, you cannot be the only eyes and ears.

HOME SECURITY

Many people live their lives with the simple belief that they will continue to live in the lifestyle that they are currently enjoying with very little thought of the future changes they may experience as they age. Some middle-aged adults think ahead, evidenced by regularly weeding out ma-

terial possessions and making the move to downsize to a more manageable home earlier rather than later when it is harder to do physically and
emotionally. However, it's just as likely that you are dealing with senior
parents who still live in your childhood home. It may be far bigger than
they reasonably need or can manage. A decision to move to a smaller
place such as senior residence or condo may be practical, but for some
families, there is just as much resistance to leaving that beloved home as
there may be to having a caregiver. It may be in the family's overall plan
to find a smaller home or apartment, but you may have to put that on the
back burner while you deal with the immediate need for home care.

Wherever they call home, it must be secured before or as soon as
reasonably possible to having employee caregivers come to the house in
an ongoing way. Unfortunately, the decision for home care can happen
rapidly and it is difficult to handle all of the preparation simultaneously.
You will just have to take the steps for home security as quickly as you
can manage. Just don't get lulled into thinking that you really don't have
to worry about it. You do.

Some of the steps for making the home itself less vulnerable are relatively simple and we will outline them here:

- Do a photographic inventory of valuables. Insurance companies
  recommend that for your most valuable items, take photos and
  make specific written descriptions:[1] save any appraisals or receipts.
  For other personal property, take photos of each room, including
  the contents of drawers and closets. Do a video walk through of the
  entire home and narrate what and where belongings are. This would
  be a great job to delegate to a pre-teen or adolescent grandchild
  because they usually have had a lot of practice with digital media.
  Make sure that your photos and videos are duplicated and stored
  with a secure system, such as a cloud service. Put it on your calendar to check and compare your photos to the actual home on a
  regular basis.
- Put the most precious family jewelry, documents (a written inventory of the home or a flash drive with the photo inventory, deeds, but
  never the only copy of the will or medical advance directives), and
  small valuables in a safe deposit box at your bank. We have heard
  many a sad story of lost family heirlooms when dementia is involved and, of course, theft.

- A fireproof safe can be a great asset and need not be too big. Documents such as those that would be used on a regular basis by an elder but that need protection such as photo ID, social security card, and insurance cards would be safely stored.[2]
- Put a deadbolt lock on the outside of a closet that only you have the code or key to. Use this for larger valuables or documents that you need immediate access to, not just during banking hours.
- Think about how the caregiver will get into the home every day. Is the elder able to answer the door? We cringe to tell you this, but we know some seniors who leave their doors unlocked for the caregiver every day. Combination door locks are available to input numerous codes for individual caregivers. Individual codes can be easily removed, but require that a reliable noncaregiver is available to add and delete codes in a timely manner. Thankfully, there are now remote access combination locks, so that from afar you can set locks to be opened by combination only at specific times, as well as delete and add codes remotely. You can receive a message when people with certain codes arrive and unlock the door and when the battery is running low.

A not so simple but essential concern regarding safety is the presence of firearms in the home. No matter what your views are on guns and gun control, guns and dementia are a potentially dangerous combination. Some adult children are afraid to visit their elderly parents who own guns for fear that they might mistake them for an intruder.[3] However, many home care agencies require that all firearms be removed from the home in order to send their employees there for caregiving. This can give families some leverage with an either/or proposition: either you let me take your guns to a safe place away from your home while you are getting home care or you can move into the nursing home where they also won't let you keep guns. While there have been tragedies of frail elderly people with guns killing innocent people, it is also a protection for the elder.[4] Elders have the highest rate of suicide by firearms.

CAMERAS: THE HIGH-TECH EYES AND EARS

We discussed in chapter 2 a number of new technologies that can be incorporated into the array of strategies to care for an elder living at home. When money is no object, there are any number of complete home security systems that can be professionally installed that include sensors and/or cameras in every conceivable nook and cranny of any home, inside and out. Some of these systems are designed specifically with seniors in mind. In some parts of Canada, the cost of a senior surveillance system has been subsidized by the local government as it is seen as a more cost-effective solution than placement in a skilled care setting.[5] For those that are handy, many home cameras have come down in price, can be viewed on one's smartphone anywhere, and are more easily set up by the consumer. These camera systems offer remote access, recording, night vision, and a two-way audio microphone that allows you to communicate with the people near the camera.[6]

We'd like to focus on cameras as they are often at the center of home security systems. They are obviously very valuable in the advancement of home security in that they provide the ability to be a witness to the activities in your elder's home. There are many instances in which this resource alone has revealed to a family when an elder is having a medical episode and needs help or when an abusive or criminal caregiver has violated the trust we place in them. Video footage from these systems is now being used by more states and is accepted as court evidence to put criminals in jail.[7]

However, cameras are intrusive, and many seniors will balk at the invasion of their privacy. It may be the answer to your dilemma, but may also feel creepy and insensitive to them. Some camera systems, such as WatchBot,[8] are designed for seniors specifically and have a feature that allows the senior to turn off the camera when they choose to. This makes more sense for an independent elder who lives alone without a caregiver. It negates the purpose, however, for someone who has care from a caregiver who could also easily deactivate it.

Discussing the purpose of the camera with your elder family member is crucial. If a person has an employed caregiver, the purpose of the camera is to monitor the care, not the elder. If you stress the importance of this device as a protective measure for your family member and they have an understanding of the inherent risks to their personal belongings and personal safety, they may wholeheartedly agree. Remind them that in any other workplace setting, an employee would have on-site supervision. Because of the unusual home setting, the caregiver should have this additional supervision to enhance the quality of care.

If you do go all in for a camera monitoring system, who is going to be monitoring the video? When? For how long? Every day? All day? The intrusive nature of the camera can go both ways. Some people will simply say that they cannot commit to such an undertaking and that is perfectly reasonable. Others insist on it. However, if you choose to go this route, realize that you will need to set some parameters for yourself as well. If you can share this duty with other family members, you will reduce some of the fatigue and stress on yourself.

RED FLAGS OF ABUSE

The vast majority of caregivers are decent, honest, and hardworking individuals. They would share your shock and disgust at the stories of abuse of elders. However, a relevant comparison can be made here to purchasing insurance: you do so to protect yourself against an adverse event. The same principle applies here. Although much of what we recommend will seem excessive, it is critical to be prepared, aware, and responsive.

This is a difficult chapter to read because it is very depressing to learn of the types and degree of abuse that vulnerable people experience. Consider these examples of headlines about elder abuse:

- "Caught on Camera: A Caregiver Abuses a 94 Year Old Woman"[9]
- "Elder Abuse Caught on Tape, Mission Viejo, CA"[10]
- "Shocking Video from Nursing Home Shows Abuse of Elderly Patient"[11]

Even a cursory search on the Internet reveals the staggering quantity of abuse that the elderly are subjected to on a daily basis.[12] We will not recount the horror stories here, but you may go to websites listed in our notes to read and watch videos of specific incidents.

We want you to be armed with the knowledge of the reality and the possibility of abuse. Know what to look for and do not hesitate to notify the authorities if you see suspicious signs. The following is from the

National Center on Elder Abuse.[13] As they say, "elder abuse can occur anywhere—in the home, in nursing homes, or other institutions. It affects seniors across all socioeconomic groups, cultures, and races."

The NCEA's Red Flags of Abuse

Neglect:

- Lack of basic hygiene, adequate food, or clean and appropriate clothing
- Lack of medical aids (glasses, walker, teeth, hearing aid, medications)
- Person with dementia left unsupervised
- Person confined to bed is left without care
- Home cluttered, filthy, in disrepair, or having fire and safety hazards
- Home without adequate facilities (stove, refrigerator, heat, cooling, working plumbing, and electricity)
- Untreated pressure "bed" sores (pressure ulcers)

Financial Abuse/Exploitation: See the next section on Financial Protection in which we go into greater detail.

Psychological/Emotional Abuse:

- Unexplained or uncharacteristic changes in behavior, such as withdrawal from normal activities or unexplained changes in alertness
- Caregiver isolates elder (doesn't let anyone into the home or speak to the elder)
- Caregiver is verbally aggressive or demeaning, controlling, overly concerned about spending money, or uncaring

Physical/Sexual Abuse:

- Inadequately explained fractures, bruises, welts, cuts, sores, or burns
- Unexplained sexually transmitted diseases

Furthermore, the NCEA has found that certain older adults are more at risk for being victims of abuse than others. Those at highest risk are:

- Women
- The very old
- People who are more isolated
- People who have dementia
- People who have mental health problems or substance abuse problems; this is the case both for the victim or the abuser (another good reason for random drug screening post-hire)

SPEAKING OF SUBSTANCE ABUSE . . .

Authorities dealing with elder abuse and exploitation have had an overwhelming increase in volume of cases related to the theft of prescription narcotics from seniors in the last decade. In addition to narcotics, thieves also seek drugs prescribed for sleep, anxiety, and depression. [14] There are stories reflecting that just about anyone who interacts with an elder in the home could be stealing medications (family members, CNAs, even hospice nurses). What can elders and families do to reduce the chance of being targeted for this frightening consequence of the drug epidemic?

- Highly sought after drugs such as prescription pain relievers should not be left in the medicine cabinet. That home safe or locked closet that was discussed earlier in the chapter would be a good storage place.
- Count these medications and keep track of them. Put out only enough of these particular drugs for the shortest time period possible. If a caregiver reports that some Percocet were dropped accidentally in the garbage and that more are needed, take note.
- Do not order refills of these drugs in advance. Most pharmacists are on the lookout for early reorders. You may not realize until you speak to the pharmacist that a caregiver has been calling to reorder without your knowledge.
- If you do not use these drugs and have overstock, call your pharmacist to find out if they have a system to dispose of them. We have seen seniors hang on to all sorts of meds from decades past; many

people raised during the Depression abhor waste of any kind, especially expensive medications. Please discuss the potential hazards, the unlikelihood of taking old prescriptions, and improved safety with disposing of them. Better they be destroyed than stay in your home as a magnet for crime.

- Before disposing of empty prescription medicine containers, tear off or black out any identifying information or refill numbers.

FINANCIAL PROTECTION

Financial exploitation of the elderly is a sad and tragic reality. According to Truelink Financial, losses for seniors have been greatly underestimated, with losses coming closer to $36.48 billion per year. [15] Ninety percent of financial exploitation occurs at the hands of family members and trusted others. [16]

The potential for this type of abuse exists when a caregiver comes into the home. We have seen it in our personal lives and in our work. However, there are steps you can take to mitigate the possibility that this may occur. We understand that it can be difficult to approach what is expected to be a caring and trusting situation by planning for the worst, but it must be done.

Financial abuse of an elder can take many forms from very small, seemingly insignificant gestures to grand larceny and identity theft. What are the potential ways in which a caregiver can take advantage of an elder to whom they have been entrusted care? Stealing, forging checks, accepting cash or check "gifts," using a credit card for personal purchases, taking material gifts, even signing over the deed to a home, car, or other personal property can happen in any setting, including assisted living and nursing homes.

Risk cannot be eliminated entirely, but there are some common sense steps you can take:

- Do an estate plan with an elder law attorney. In the process of this planning, you or another family member can assume financial power of attorney should the need arise. Knowing where and how assets are distributed will help later in monitoring the financial situation should the need occur. Identify and make careful notes of bank, retirement, and other accounts. Make multiple copies of all legal documents and provide those copies to other trusted family members.

- If possible, especially in the case of particularly vulnerable elders who have dementia, forward all mail to your address or a PO box. Even after making this request, expect that banks and other institutions may continue to send copies to an elder's home address due to computer systems that govern address changes. If your family member is willing, take over bill paying so you can see firsthand any activity on accounts.
- If you are using an agency or online company, ask about specific company policies regarding accusations against caregivers and the limits of their liability insurance. If a caregiver is taking an elder out to eat or shop, how are funds used and accounted for?
- Realize that vulnerable elders will often hide the fact that a caregiver is asking for and receiving money. You will need to rely on careful monitoring of accounts to detect irregularities.
- If you are hiring someone not affiliated with a business, you absolutely must purchase insurance to protect your elder's estate from lawsuit. Check with your insurance agent on the best type of policy to purchase for this coverage.

Now that your due diligence is complete, what are the signs of financial exploitation?

- Withdrawals of money inconsistent with older person's spending habits
- Withdrawals of money inconsistent with older person's income
- Will, property title, or valuable asset bequeathed to "new" beneficiary
- Older person "can't find" or "misplaced" valuable personal belongings
- Unusual credit card activity or new credit card account
- Lack of necessities or amenities older person can afford
- Unfilled prescriptions or untreated medical problems
- Caregiving incommensurate with older person's income. For example, a caregiver strongly suggests additional hours of care that aren't supported by need.

- Documents missing like insurance policies, credit card statements, medical reports, or any other paperwork that has identifying information on it
- Suspicious signature on documents
- Financial documents altered
- Caregiver takes up residence with the older person (this is much more likely with a nonagency caregiver). We have seen instances in which a "trusted" caregiver moves in with the elder under the guise of ease of caretaking duties, with the real purpose being financial exploitation.
- Mail redirected
- Prepaid packages missing
- Incessant phone calls from caregiver. Most agencies will not permit caregivers to call a client directly and should this happen, contact the agency. If the behavior persists, there could be a problem and the situation needs to be looked into further.[17]

Financial Fraud Alert: Beware the Telephone

As we have mentioned in an earlier chapter, the phone line has special significance for seniors. There is so much history and memory involved for an older person and their telephone. Not only has it literally been a line to the outside world for most of their life, for many it continues to be the preferred communication technology over more recent devices such as a smartphone or the Internet. For the older generation, there is a certain telephone etiquette that is perhaps missing today in the world of cell phones. Many older people are in the habit of being polite on the phone and would think it is very rude to hang up on anyone.[18] In addition, many elders are isolated, bored, and lonely and may feel hopeful any time the phone rings. A special kind of criminal knows all these things. Combine that with the older generation's well-known good habits of savings and thrift and they become a favorite target for scammers and thieves who realize there are likely to be funds of some kind to plunder.

You are probably familiar with the typical and pervasive calls and scams: the robocall that announces "your credit card account is at risk—answer now"; the person acting as a police authority who is calling to say "your grandson got pulled over in Mexico and needs you to bail him out today for $5,000!"; someone pretending to call from the bank, the utility company, or another recognized institution asking for an update to your account, "now if you would please tell us your social security number for verification." They know how to sound authentic and are friendly and take all the time in the world with a vulnerable senior to fleece them.

Some financial fraud experts advise getting rid of landline phones.[19] However, depending on the elder needing care, manual dexterity and vision could be limited and the required learning curve for a smartphone could eliminate this as a viable option. There are some smartphones designed for seniors with bigger numbers and touch pads to reduce dialing error. One solution may be if you or your elder have a caregiver, they can assist in screening calls. This needs to be a discussion with you, your elder family member, and the caregiver. Some elders may resent the need for anyone helping them screen calls, especially if dementia of any level is present. Some caregivers think that it is none of their business to tell their client who they can or cannot talk to on the phone. They do not want to be disrespectful. Their care agency may have a protocol for phone calls that you may not be aware of, so you need to connect with the supervisor too. Make sure to have a three- or four-way conversation so that everyone is on the same page to prevent financial fraud on the phone.

HOW TO ASSESS COMPLAINTS ABOUT A CAREGIVER

Every caregiver situation is different and it is critical to evaluate complaints from an elder in the context of their ability to accurately convey what is going on. If someone has full awareness and the capacity to express and describe their circumstances, you will likely take their complaints at face value. However, if your elder has dementia, it may be more complicated to assess what the true reality of the situation is. In our work, we have observed countless times when an elder states, "My wedding ring is missing! That awful caregiver stole it!" If you have done your inventory and know that the ring is safe and sound, how do you address these complaints and what do they mean? Here are some suggestions:

- Take every complaint about a caregiver seriously. At least in the beginning. Some elders will never accept a caregiver in their home and there will be an inevitable roller coaster of acceptance one day and rejection the next.

- Check in frequently to ask how things are going. Many elders will be reluctant to "get someone in trouble" by expressing frustration or problems with a caregiver.
- If you are in the same town, take the time to sit down and talk with your elder about any problem. Listen and acknowledge their concerns. Are there accusations of stealing, verbal abuse, or neglect? If you are unable to meet face to face, ask a friend or other family member, care manager, or supervisor at the agency to assess the situation.
- Report the problem to the agency or state authorities if appropriate. (More about how to do this later in the chapter.)
- Accept that a complaint may mean the caregiver is not a good fit or is simply a poor caregiver. Request a change. However, if multiple caregivers come and go and the grievances continue, then the problem is most likely not the caregivers themselves.
- Repetitious complaints of stealing that you are certain have no basis in reality can be very frustrating to deal with. You and the agency will have to accept that this is likely to be ongoing and can't be resolved. That is why it is critical to have completed the inventory and put into place all of the safeguards we have suggested.

Paul's Story

Paul is an eighty-five-year-old man who has been diagnosed with Alzheimer's disease. He lives in his own home and over time has required more and more assistance to take care of basic daily tasks. His family convinces him to try a caregiver. Having been a "ladies man" his whole life, he agrees to have two female caregivers assist him during the week with cooking, cleaning, laundry, and medication reminders. One caregiver works Monday through Thursday and the other one Friday through Sunday. Paul's persona takes on a new and somewhat troubling form due to his cognitive impairment. He begins to talk about "marrying" one of the caregivers and refers to her as his "girlfriend" in public. Hugs become more frequent with an occasional pat on the bottom, which is gently discouraged by the caregiver.

Paul and the caregiver often go out to eat and shop for groceries and clothes with funds provided by his family on a weekly basis. As time goes on, Paul starts to buy the caregiver's meals when they are out to eat.

This progresses to buying gas for her car when she transports him and soon thereafter she is asking Paul for cash saying she will "pay it back," all the while encouraging his misplaced affections to further ensure his continued financial support. Paul's family becomes suspicious when they notice that Paul is running out of money sooner and asking for more. Paul's family talks to him about the situation and he readily admits that he had been giving money to the caregiver. The agency confronts the caregiver about the situation and she says that she had been accepting money, but that Paul "insisted" on giving it to her.

As you read Paul's story you may be thinking to yourself, "That's not so serious. No harm was done." Make no mistake, what was done by this caregiver is classified as financial exploitation and was also against the agency's policies and procedures. Exploitation can start small and get much, much bigger. Care providers who become exploiters and thieves don't necessarily start out this way. Many rationalize a small infraction due to some negative event in their lives by saying to themselves "well, just this once" or "I really deserve this." Then the situation starts to spiral out of control, gain severity, and become an accepted habit.

Circle of Friends

Many adult children of elders live out of state and are unable to take the kind of hands-on approach we talk about here. Don't worry, we have some suggestions on how to create a circle of friends, or in some cases professionals, to be your eyes and ears. Monitoring a caregiving situation is part of the larger responsibility to advocate and protect your family member. You may be reluctant to ask others to assume this responsibility, but defining the role will help other people understand and appreciate what is expected. If you are asking a friend, other family members, a church member, or someone else in the community to check in with your elder, we suggest the following:

- Make the drop in visits time limited. Ask someone to drop in once a week or every other week if that is the most they can do.
- Be specific. Let the person know what to look for. For example, ask them to look in the fridge, check the home for cleanliness, talk to the elder, and take a close look at their hygiene and overall health status.

- Ask for a report by e-mail, if possible, as soon after the visit as possible. That way you have a written record.
- Most people are reluctant to report on something that they think they have no expertise in. In our work, we have come to trust our "gut" when it comes to detecting things that just don't seem right.
- If you have the financial resources, consider hiring a geriatric care manager who can monitor and manage the situation on a regular basis.

Expand Your Circle

Many elders have a village of helpers. This includes home health personnel (physical and occupational therapists, nurses, and aides), housekeepers, dog walkers, and any number of other people who come to the home on a regular basis. These people can be an excellent source of information on how things are going. You can even hire professional senior care auditors to check on the care of your elder. For example, Penrose Senior Care Auditors (https://penroseseniorcareauditors.com/), serving thirty states, allows you to choose the level of check in by a professional senior care auditor and receive a report on their findings of the level of care in the home. This is not a geriatric care manager service. Rather, it is a service to make drop-by visits to witness and review what care is happening and report back to you. You can arrange for as many or as few visits as you want.

A person's physician can be an excellent source of information about a caregiver situation. Sometimes an elder will feel much more comfortable talking to their physician than with you. As long as you have health-care power of attorney and permission to talk with the physician, make sure you get regular updates on visits if you can't attend.

If you suspect things aren't going well, don't hesitate to ask other helpers what their impressions are. They may have noticed a change in behavior or observed something troubling about a caregiver and just don't feel like it is their place to mention it. Older people often form close and trusting relationships with these "helpers" and they can be an invaluable source of information.

Don't Let Denial Cloud Your Vision

Denial is a human tendency that we all have at one time or another. In some instances, it can be very helpful to allow us to continue to persevere and survive in spite of overwhelming realities. According the Merriam-Webster dictionary, denial is "a psychological defense mechanism in which confrontation with a personal problem or with reality is avoided by denying the existence of the problem or reality."[20] We can be in denial that our diet has gone off the tracks when we make a habit of eating a six-hundred-calorie blueberry muffin loaded with sugar every day. Further, we can use rationalization (another defensive thought process) when we decide to see the daily muffin as a health food because it has fruit in it.

When it comes to our relationships and safety, however, denial can be a serious problem. It is usually involved when there is little time to step back and carefully consider all the facets of what you are observing or feeling about a situation. Here are some suggestions for turning your denial into a tool to help you prevent yourself or your elder family member from being taken advantage of:

- Recognize your denial thoughts. Consider your response to a parent's numerous complaints about how a caregiver is "going through all the drawers in the house," but the caregiver is telling you that she is just tidying up a couple of overstuffed drawers with your parent supervising. You might have the thought, "Those drawers have needed cleaning out for years. I'll just wait and see how this turns out; I don't have time to deal with this now, it's probably not as bad as mom thinks it is." The key denial thought here is the time pressure and wanting to fend off having to think about it more. These thoughts can prevent you from following up when you need to.

- Be aware that your relationship with and your feelings for the caregiver can also play powerfully into thoughts of denial. Once your family has established a good rapport with a caregiver, you have experience with their good care, and you begin to know them as a person, you feel gratitude and caring. If something comes up that seems suspicious, it may be your first inclination to think, "Well, of course Mary Ann would not have purchased groceries for herself when she was shopping with mom. They just must have been stocking up, because it seems like they spent enough to feed a family of four." Your fond feelings, appreciation, and loyalty for the caregiver can interfere with a rational assessment of the situation.

- Listen to your feelings. Do you have a feeling of discomfort when you hear an explanation from a caregiver of some unusual finding or happenings in the home? Say your mother with moderate dementia has gone with the caregiver to the bank to take out $20 in cash a time or two more than usual for the month. The caregiver says, "Oh, you know your mother, she gets really anxious if there isn't a certain amount of cash in her wallet. She got really upset with me when I told her that we already did that last week. So I took her so she could take a little out and she would be calm. Then she wanted to go to the drugstore to buy some toiletries. Would you rather we call you if it happens again?" On the surface, it may sound reasonable, especially when you are planning a presentation for work and have many other things on your mind. You may think, "Sure, I guess mom has sort of been that way. Let her spend her money on whatever she wants." But that lingering feeling of doubt and discomfort is sometimes your best indicator that something is wrong.
- Find a sounding board. When you recognize that you may have some denial thoughts and ongoing feelings of discomfort, it's time to speak your concerns out loud. Talk to a family member or friend to share your concerns. They may be able to give you some valuable feedback about your response. They may even be able to help you check on the situation. They may know you well enough to know that you tend to believe the goodness in everyone no matter what or know if you tend to let certain things slide when others don't.

HOW TO REPORT SUSPECTED ABUSE OR EXPLOITATION

After you have gone beyond feeling suspicious and possibly have confirmation or evidence that something criminal could be going on at your parent's home, do not hesitate to call for help. First and foremost, if there is any sense of physical danger to yourself or your family member, call the police. The police will likely take your report, investigate any criminal activity, and refer you to Adult Protective Services for further help.

Please note if you have hired through an agency: of course you must contact them and tell the administrators at the agency. But do not let that stop you from directly reporting criminal behavior to the authorities. Here is how to contact these resources:

- Call 911 or the local police for any imminent physical danger
- Call Eldercare Locator at 1-800-677-1116 or go to eldercare.gov
- For the state numbers for Adult Protective Services, go to www.apsnetwork.org or visit the National Center on Elder Abuse's website, www.ncea.aoa.gov

Adult Protective Services (APS) are state and local agencies that are available in every state in the United States. In general terms, APS provides protective services to elderly and vulnerable adults eighteen years old and older, much like Child Protective Services intervene on behalf of children. In most states, APS is under the administration of social services, but other states may have APS under the management of a department of aging or health. APS responds to reports that involve any type of elder abuse, including financial exploitation and fraud, physical abuse, sexual abuse, neglect, and self-neglect. Self-neglect is a special category of behavior sometimes seen in the elderly population. It is indicated when older adults do not take care of themselves when they appear to have the ability to do so, such as refusing help or assistance and then having injury or illness as a result. We will look at self-neglect in more detail in chapter 6. States vary on reporting requirements of suspected abuse, neglect, and exploitation. All states have "mandatory reporting requirements," some of which require anyone who suspects abuse to report it to Adult Protective Services.

As with many public services these days, APS has suffered due to seemingly unending budget cuts common in many states. According to a survey by the National Association of Adult Protective Services Administrators in 2003, most states reported that APS agencies are underfunded and understaffed, in some cases having very limited authority and their restricted resources limit them in finding appropriate shelter for abuse victims who need to be removed from a residence.[21] Over our combined careers in geriatric care, we have seen a decrease in the ability of local APSs in several states to respond quickly to reports of suspicious activity involving elders. Sometimes there is a long wait before a person is seen and assessed, unless there is concern about immediate physical safety. It has become such a concern that in some places, health professionals do not even want to report to APS because they do not have confidence in the response even though they have a professional duty to report.[22]

Families also hesitate to report. One family we knew a number of years ago had hired a caregiver to make a daily visit to assist the husband in taking his blood pressure medication. He had had a stroke and this medication was essential. He also had moderate dementia and could not reliably remember to take the daily dose. His wife, who had no problems with remembering, had advanced arthritis and other physical limitations and could not manage to give the pills to her husband. While the couple had these limitations, they otherwise enjoyed living in their own condo in their same neighborhood and near their longtime doctors. The adult children all lived out of town, so on the recommendation of a friend, they hired this particular friendly caregiver to drop by daily to give the medication. At first, all seemed well. The caregiver and the wife reported that the arrangement was helpful and the couple enjoyed the brief company of the caregiver. The adult children sent a regular check to the caregiver. Months later, their mother admitted that they hardly ever saw the caregiver and that the medications were rarely given. When the children called the friend who had also hired the same caregiver, they found out that they had had a similar experience and had evidence that the caregiver was stealing from their parent. The friend urged the family to report to APS and the police. The family declined, saying that they did not want to embarrass their parents any further. In fact, they were making arrangements to move their parents to a facility near them in another state.

In spite of the huge caseload and constant referrals of new elders in need of assessment, APS is a resource to provide information to you and help you sort out what needs to be done to stop the abuse from happening. Even if you are uncertain, a call to APS can help clarify what needs to be done to protect a vulnerable person. In some states, your identity will not be shared if you report suspected abuse. The assessment of APS can assist the criminal investigation and prosecution of a perpetrator.

One surprising challenge that APS often faces is when an elder shares information about the illegal activity of someone who is supposed to be caring for them and then says that they do not want to proceed with an investigation. The elder may feel shame for having been a victim, concern about hurting someone who has at some point helped them, or have rationalized that they somehow deserved the abuse or that no one else will help them if they get this person in trouble. (This refuting of a previous statement is most often when the abuser is a family member, but it does also happen with paid caregivers.)

If you can prepare yourself and your family member for the potentially long process involved in reporting to social services and for the legal system to assist you, you can then decide to make a commitment to following through if it becomes a criminal case. When good evidence exists, it can be a relatively quick process. Knowing that your reporting can protect you from further harm and could prevent someone else from being abused by the same caregiver can be incentive for many.

There are promising trends in different parts of the United States that may help prevent elder abuse and prosecute criminal caregivers more effectively. States are passing legislation making it a crime to financially exploit adults who are cognitively impaired.[23] Some states around the country have an Adult Abuse Registry so that consumers and law enforcement can look up a potential caregiver to see if they have any history of this type of crime. Perhaps one of the best changes being considered in some states is the combining of APS with law enforcement. When law enforcement officers who are specially trained to understand the nuances of elder abuse are designated to work together with APS in an ongoing way, the results could be more effective care and prosecution. Many states are forming task forces to prevent financial predators from targeting the elderly and working with financial institutions to add safety nets for their vulnerable customers. All of these efforts are necessary to protect our most vulnerable adults. In the meantime, we must continue to watch out for our elder family members the best that we can.

INTERVIEW WITH AN APS INVESTIGATOR

Have you had a situation that you've had to investigate that involved a hired caregiver caring for an elderly person who financially exploited that person? If so, could you give a brief description of what occurred and what the outcome was?

I have investigated many financial exploitation cases where the caregiver has exploited the victim. Very often there is money, medication, or personal belongings that disappear. Some of these items can be very valuable. Often the victim has limited mental capacity and it is difficult to prove that the caregiver took the item or if the victim misplaced it or hid it or if a family member took it for safekeeping or to have it themselves. It is often difficult to prove the caretaker was the perpetrator or which caretaker was the perpetrator. Sometimes there are a lot of people in and out of the home and many times family members seem to be the likely perpetrator. Many cases are closed as inconclusive due to these unknown factors.

I worked a case where the caregiver became such a good friend and advocate for the elderly woman the caregiver had her change her trust and put them on as the beneficiary to her home and all of her assets. On this case the victim and the perpetrator had a falling out and everything was changed back. Sometimes the victims feel so much more support from the perpetrator that they are very open about how their children do nothing for them and they don't want anything left to them and want some person or organization to inherit whatever they have left when they die.

I see caregivers asking for loans frequently and due to the friendship they have with the victims, they frequently want to help them out and pay for their car to be fixed or help their son pay off fines or whatever. I think sometimes the victims feel obligated to help. These perpetrators see them at very vulnerable times like when they are showering and home all alone.

What is a typical day like for you?

A typical day for me is coming into the office in the morning and opening any new cases that I got the prior day. Then I do all the paperwork to close any cases. I return and make telephone calls to referents and collateral contacts. In the later morning or early afternoon I go into the field and investigate. I try not to do too many field investigations in one day because then it takes the next day to document everything I did and it can get overwhelming documenting for hours. Some days I don't leave my office because there is so much documentation to be done. I try to do a good blend of paperwork and field visits each day.

What is the most challenging part of your job?

The most challenging aspect of my job is wanting to do more for the victims but there are not services for them. We investigate and don't do any case management. We refer to basic community resources and then close the case. I hate to see the victims of scams. They have often lost thousands of dollars, sometimes mortgaging their house and cars to get money to send to out-of-country scammers and there is nothing I can do for them but document what happened. It is a tragedy. Many times law enforcement do not want to work with our victims and seem to have more important things to investigate or follow up on than what we refer to them. If the same things were happening to a child or an animal, people would be outraged. Many victims see APS as someone who is finally there to help them. It is frustrating when we can't help them solve the issue and they are left in the same situation still vulnerable to future abuse, neglect, or exploitation.

Another aspect of the job that is hard is that I never know what happens to the perpetrators. I know that very few are criminally prosecuted. Once I close the case and refer it to law enforcement I never hear if the case was dropped or followed through with or what. I am never called to be a witness in court and rarely do police officers need anything from me, which makes me wonder what happens to the cases that are supported by APS and given to law enforcement.

There are also in-house pressures to see victims within a certain time frame and to close cases within so many days. I fear that these time frames become more important than improving a person's life. I often wonder if what I do makes a difference.

TAKEAWAY POINTS FOR THIS CHAPTER

- Secure the home by doing an appropriate inventory of valuables and moving those valuables to more secure locations.
- Consider how the caregiver will get into the home and put in a front door lock with the ability to add and delete codes for entry.
- Camera systems can offer many advantages but are also intrusive. Be sure to discuss the purpose of having them with the elder for their protection.
- Though we hope that you never have the experience, be aware and alert to all the types of elder abuse that happen.
- Meet with an elder estate planning attorney to do an estate plan that may include financial power of attorney. If you are making plans for a family member, make certain you bring them with you!
- Ask for permission to have all mail forwarded to a PO box or your personal address.
- Ask for permission to monitor financial accounts and possibly assume bill paying duties.
- Recognized the signs of financial exploitation.
- Identify a "circle of friends" to assist you in monitoring the situation and call on them when necessary.
- Have a plan of action to contact authorities if you do need to report elder abuse.

6

YOUR HOME, YOUR CARE

Though the care agency websites and advertising brochures may lure you into thinking that most seniors are happy and carefree when they have a hired caregiver helping them in their home, it is not an easy adjustment for most. A primary reason that elders struggle with getting assistance is how we as a society view the core idea of independence. In this chapter we will discuss what that means for individuals psychologically and as a part of aging. Appreciating how independence and dependence play a role in the success or failure of an elder person's experience with ongoing personal care will help you design a better fit.

The concept of independence throughout one's adult life is an ideal that shapes our attitudes about aging. Once a person emerges from adolescence (and sometimes before), we fully expect them (as adults) to be self-reliant and autonomous for the remainder of their lifetime. Not only do we believe this, our laws confirm and uphold our rights in this regard except under unusual circumstances. The ideal of independence is shaped by experience.

THE MAKING OF AN AGING ERA

Personal characteristics of a generation can't be separated from the historical context in which they grew up. Understanding how someone's values and beliefs were formed can help to explain not only their current decisions, but their expectations, what they believe is important, and ultimately how they age. Each era has its unique challenges, opportunities, and values. People born between approximately 1910 and the 1920s are often referred to as the "greatest generation," a phrase coined by Tom Brokaw in his book *The Greatest Generation.* These individuals are in their late eighties and nineties now. Some are one hundred years old or older. People born between roughly 1925 and 1945 are referred to as the "silent generation." These individuals are in their seventies and eighties.

The greatest generation endured the Great Depression and went through World War II. The characteristics and values generally ascribed to them are pride in personal responsibility, thriftiness, a strong work ethic, savers, and self-reliant. You can see where this is going . . . who doesn't have a story of grandma keeping thousands of dollars' worth of cash in various places in her house, refusing to buy anything new because what she has "will do," foregoing necessities because they simply are not viewed as being, well, necessary. Doing without was a mantra for many of this generation because they had to survive on so little, never knowing if or when the sacrifice would end.

The silent generation is those folks born between 1925 and 1945. They too grew up with war and economic instability. The traits most commonly associated with them are a trust in government, humbleness, striving quietly for economic success, patriotic, and being nonrebellious. These admirable traits are the very ones that make this generation and the one before it trusting and therefore vulnerable to exploitation. Moreover, these older adults are loath to receive help, believing in the self-reliance that defines their generation. This self-reliance and "bootstrap" mentality is what helped them survive during extremely stressful times. Understanding these values can help to explain the resistance to accepting help from others.

The traits of older adults today are generally a strong work ethic, saving and not spending on what isn't necessary, placing great emotional value in home, and a strong belief that people take care of their own problems. A fierce independence was formed during a time of extreme strife and sacrifice and also a quiet humility and trust in humanity. Many older people of both of these generations own their own homes, have savings, and possibly have a pension from working for the same company for decades.

Judith's Story

Judith is an eighty-five-year-old widowed woman who lives alone in her own home. She has slowed down over the years due to a heart arrhythmia, scoliosis that she has had since she was a teenager, and the beginning of macular degeneration. Her family has urged her to accept private caregiving in the home to assist with tasks like cooking, driving, and cleaning. Judith has resisted these suggestions despite the fact that she has a long-term care policy that might qualify her for these services. She and Jim bought the policy decades ago and have paid nearly $200,000 so far in premiums. But Judith says, "I don't think I am ready yet for help. I am able to do everything I need to and I don't want anyone else coming into my home." Hearing about Judith's early years may help to understand her independent spirit.

During Judith's early twenties she, like so many women, was living at home until the war ended in 1945. Pretty much the only jobs single women pursued were teaching or nursing. Judith met a young man, Jim, just out of the service, and they married and began a life together. Those early years were lean. Jim went to college on the GI Bill while Judith worked cleaning houses, doing secretarial work, and babysitting. They started a family. Their living situation was basically one apartment after the other, including a room in the back of someone's house where they shared a bathroom and had a hotplate and sink. Eventually they lived in student housing, which consisted of row after row of identical metal structures. Judith says in those days it was not unusual for wives to take jobs to support their husbands going to school.

When Jim graduated he went from job to job trying to find something satisfying yet stable while Judith learned to make the few dollars they had last until the next paycheck. To keep track of what money they had, Jim and Judith came up with a system of putting cash in various envelopes labeled rent, utilities, and food. Canned beans became the staple at the end of the month when they were waiting for another paycheck. Jim eventually landed a position with General Electric, which brought some much-needed financial stability. Judith had learned to make their money last, and that did not change with Jim's better paying job. Eventually they were able to buy a house through the GI Bill and Judith says, "We bought one of the Levittown homes in the suburbs which was less expensive than continuing to rent."[1] Judith and Jim had three children altogether during these more prosperous times, but Judith states that they paid by cash or check for everything and the idea of "owing" money was irresponsible. You paid for what you could afford.

Judith's story tells us much about this generation—their hardships and patterns of saving, hard work, and sacrificing for their families, and the idea that you work for what you have and spend wisely.

AGING LONGER

The average lifespan for a male born in 1900 was forty-seven years. In 2016 life expectancy is about seventy-nine years of age. Years ago families took care of elders often with several generations living under one roof. Today families often live in an entirely different part of the country, and as Atul Gawande says in his book *Being Mortal: Medicine and What Matters in the End*, "old age and infirmity have gone from being a shared, multi-generational responsibility to a more or less private state—something experienced largely alone or with the aid of doctors and institutions."[2]

Medical advances since 1900 are difficult to comprehend as there have been so many. The end result is that people are being kept alive longer with these medical advances, but they are not necessarily healthy as they age. There is no cure for cancer, end stage renal disease, or Alzheimer's disease, but there are interventions for all of those conditions. An article in the *Chicago Tribune* titled "We all Want to Die with Dignity—But Not Yet" stated, "Medical advances bring the promise of extending life, but some of the treatments used in a person's last months, weeks or days—such as CPR for failing hearts, dialysis for failing kidneys and feeding tubes for those unable to nourish themselves—often do not provide more time and can worsen quality of life."[3] In our experience it is often family members, not the elders themselves, who insist upon medical interventions that will neither prolong life nor add quality to the life remaining.

As people live longer with these chronic diseases, they need more and more help. Often one event can cause a cascade of problems that can be very challenging to get a handle on, especially for family living at a distance. And as people live longer, they need the financial and family resources to provide for the care and support that they require, whether they stay at home, move to assisted living, or end up in long-term care. Despite a lifetime of savings, ownership of a home, and retirement and social security income, finances can become strained.

Baby boomers and millennials are faced with the task of caring for and making decisions for a group of aging adults who are living longer and therefore more vulnerable to the diseases and disabilities associated with age. The desire to remain at home for as long as possible while coping with many of these inevitable changes puts pressure on the resources available to make this happen.

As medical problems begin to mount, older people become more dependent. This can happen incrementally or suddenly. Dependence as an adult can be a consequence of aging that most everyone wants to avoid. When an older person who has lived his or her entire adult life as a competent adult develops a condition that threatens to change that, it is often a shock. It is not uncommon for people to react with denial, minimizing, and avoidance. That often includes the family. As a family member struggling to cope with these changes, they may be faced with their own feelings of mortality or illness. What will aging look like? Will it look like this?

THE BULL IN THE CHINA SHOP

There is nothing like a crisis to expedite poor decision making. We have all been there. Months of little safety concerns suddenly coalesce into one big event like a fall or an ER visit and something must be done! Before you become the "bull in the china shop," understand that nothing can really be done unless your senior agrees to whatever you have in mind. Making decisions "for" an elder likely brings about a mix of feelings: relief that you are able to take charge, but queasy knowing that it just doesn't feel quite right.

Multitasking is the forte of a generation of baby boomers and millennials who are juggling careers, children, and aging parents. Fixing a pressing problem quickly and efficiently is probably what you do best. Mom needs a care provider and I will just get one as soon as possible! Except that mom is being incredibly stubborn to the point of sounding like a two-year-old who only seems to know the word "no." It is crystal clear to you and other members of your family that an intervention is needed to keep mom safe, whether it be using oxygen at night, taking prescribed medications, having a caregiver in the home, using a walker, not driving—the list goes on. You have difficulty understanding how a reasonable person can make decisions that compromise their safety.

We have talked in earlier chapters about having "the talk" and ways to cope with resistance. The delicate and complicated role reversal that happens between adult children and their aging parents is at the root of many a strained and sometimes irreparable relationship. If you have children under the age of eighteen, you make decisions on their behalf because they are still considered minors. If you make decisions for another adult, regardless of their perceived inability to make good decisions, are you infringing upon their rights?

Take a step back and consider what it must be like to slowly lose friends, abilities, independence, autonomy, and control. Think about the embarrassment and shame that accompanies these losses. Sometimes saying "no" is one way to exert control over a deteriorating situation or to reassert the fact that your parent is still your parent and not a child.

The values we talked about earlier in this chapter can come into full force now with the belief that things can be managed without outside interference or help. Moreover, many seniors don't want to be a burden to their children or grandchildren. As losses mount, it can be overwhelming and depressing. In other cases, there is simply an inability for an older adult to recognize that a problem exists. This could be due to cognitive impairment like dementia or depression. Managing these situations is challenging and frustrating.

ETHICAL DILEMMAS ABOUND

The chances of living longer with a lower quality of life and at a greater cost is a troubling future for anyone to consider and is not lost on the older generation. As they draw nearer to the loss of independence and potential for disability and loss of control over decisions, some elders are putting their feet down. They want to have a say in treatment matters that may fly in the face of the wishes of family, doctors, and the law. Consider this example, as described in a *New York Times* article titled "Complexities of Choosing an End Game for Dementia."[4] Jerome Medalie, an eighty-eight-year-old spry retired lawyer, has added to his otherwise usual advance directives that should he develop dementia, all food and water are to be withheld so that it may hasten his own death. This is referred to as "voluntarily stopping eating and drinking" or VSED. This is a concept usually reserved for end-of-life discussions, not for response to a future diagnosis. He has specified that his wife will act as his health proxy and carry through with this directive should he develop this condition. It is easy to imagine all the problems that this advance directive will create. If his wife tries to carry out his wishes, will she be arrested for manslaughter or murder? What if when he actually has dementia, he forgets his plan and he protests and wishes to eat and drink? What if his wife predeceases him? Will his children be expected to follow through? And if he lives in a nursing home, assisted living facility, or lives at home with a caregiver, how could they possibly fulfill his directive? It would not only be a liability issue, it could also be a criminal case. As the rate of dementia increases due to the growing aging population, we will likely see more explicit and ethically challenging and difficult directives from the baby boomers. So many of us want to do it "our way."

As you assess your own reaction to Mr. Medalie's directive, consider that most families may not have an elder who has taken these legal steps to have it their way but have expressed their demands for control in some fashion. For example, we have talked to a family who say that they have an uncle who tells them seriously, "when I have dementia or Parkinson's, just wheel me out on the dock and roll me over the edge, okay?" Or two old gentlemen were overheard discussing a friend who had a chronic and painful disability and concluded, "well, if that happens to us, it's time to bring out the Smith & Wesson." Some may consider this suicide. Some may not and instead conclude that it is a valid choice for a rugged American individual to make. Whatever you think of it in a theoretical sense, imagine being asked to carry out this type of directive for someone you love.

Elders who push the envelope in less dramatic ways still present challenges for families. A more common scenario is an elder choosing to ignore medical advice. These issues will likely sound more familiar. As a society, we have a set of conflicting beliefs about the rights of the individual and seeking safety over risk. For example, Tom's mother is obese, diabetic, and after years of living with this chronic illness, is just plain old tired of having her insulin checked and changing insulin doses every day. She eats a gallon of ice cream at a time and her doctor has warned her of dire medical consequences. Her response? "Who cares? It's my life!" She refuses to let the caregiver check her glucose level, resulting in repeated crisis calls. Another story involves an older man who has a permanent tracheostomy. He refuses anyone who tries to do maintenance care and cleaning on his trache and has even been known to smoke a cigar through this airway. Another elder's caregiver calls his daughter frantically when he routinely refuses to wear his oxygen. You may assume that these problems could be solved by having this elder declared mentally incompetent and sending them to a skilled nursing facility. However, even if legal action is taken, these facilities may also struggle with finding immediate solutions to health-threatening behavior. The effort to get someone who is unwilling to move out of their home even if it seems the most reasonable option is in itself a complex and draining task.

We expect that we will see more of this to come, and from people who would not be candidates for being declared mentally incompetent. The next wave of elders, the baby boomers, is already preparing themselves to control their lives and lifestyle into their old age. Some have witnessed the struggle and pain of debility of their own parents and are determined not to experience the same when they reach that age. In his controversial article "Why I Hope to Die at 75,"[5] Ezekiel Emanuel, a well-known physician and author, asserts that he has no intention of suicide at that age. However, he states his case for his decision to end all medical care for himself at the age of seventy-five except for palliative care. Writing as a healthy fifty-seven-year-old, Emanuel further clarifies that he wants no more preventative care after sixty-five, such as colonoscopies, checks for prostate cancer, or flu and pneumonia vaccinations. He argues that research indicates that though Americans will live longer than their parents before them, "they are likely to be more incapacitated. Does that sound very desirable? Not to me."

The care industry thinks that it has problems now due to the shortage of good caregivers. Imagine how it will address an increasing number of aging individuals who will be asserting their demands for custom care along with ever-increasing ethical and legal minefields such as these.

DIGNITY OF RISK

The concept of "dignity of risk" was first coined during the deinstitution-alization era for people with intellectual disabilities in the 1970s.[6] The concept was intended to allow people to fail while respecting each individual's autonomy and self-determination. Robert Perske, an author and advocate of persons with intellectual disabilities, asserted that all adults lose the potential for personal growth when they are overly protected and that there is "dehumanizing indignity in safety." The disability and mental health communities have rallied around this idea as a way to promote growth and confidence by allowing people to fail.

With elders, this concept is making its way into the consciousness of the community. Even in guardianship, there is a growing movement to provide incapacitated adults with more autonomy and "person-centered planning." Person-centered planning accepts where the person is emotionally and psychologically, respecting that person's decisions about their own care and vision for the future.

Some questions to consider in making decisions for an older adult:

- Can you actually assure that someone is safe?
- When does keeping someone "safe" mean that there is too much restriction to someone's autonomy or quality of life?
- What does it mean to be safe or free from risk? Who makes this decision?

"There is risk and consequence to every choice, every aspect of life. Some persons choose to live with more risk than do others, and are willing to accept the consequences of their choices."[7] Easy to say, but not so easy to do when you are faced with a decision about how to protect someone from themselves. At what point does safety override someone's freedom to make decisions?

SUPPORTED DECISION MAKING AND GUARDIANSHIP

The idea of supported decision making can be a good way to approach a conversation with a resistant elder. One definition is: "The purpose of supported decision making is to help individuals understand the options, responsibilities, and consequences of their decisions; obtain and understand information relevant to their decisions; and communicate their decisions to the appropriate people."[8] Many of the same principles discussed in chapter 4 apply here, but it is worth repeating that despite your inclination to immediately calm the troubled waters, it is worth taking some time to think through an approach that is more likely to solve the problem rather than exacerbate it.

It is a delicate balance to avoid overprotection while acknowledging personal preferences, choices, and the dignity of risk, while at the same time setting appropriate and person-centered safeguards if at all possible. Certainly families have found themselves in situations that call for immediate action. We are not suggesting that dignity of risk be used as a rationale to avoid a crisis. In many of these cases, families may be shocked to discover that their elder is exhibiting self-neglect. Self-neglect generally means the individual neglects to attend to basic needs such as personal hygiene, nutrition, or tending appropriately to any medical conditions that they have. At times like this, a call to Adult Protected Services might be warranted, but they too have limitations to what they are authorized to do to protect an individual, and many families understandably don't want a state agency involved. Be aware, however, that some states require anyone who suspects neglect, abuse, or exploitation to report this to Adult Protective Services.

Some states only require certain professionals to report their concerns. Other states require all citizens to report their concerns. The 2013 Nationwide Survey of State Mandatory Reporting Requirements for Elderly and/or Vulnerable Persons Mandatory Reporting Chart provides reporting requirements for each state.[9]

For example, California requires the following: "Any person who has assumed full or intermittent responsibility for the care or custody of an elder or dependent adult, whether or not he or she receives compensation, including administrators, supervisors, and any licensed staff of a public or private facility that provides care or services for elder or dependent adults, or any elder or dependent adult care custodian, health practitioner, clergy member, or employee of a county adult protective services."

In contrast, Texas mandates the following: "A person having cause to believe that an elderly or disabled person is in the state of abuse, neglect, or exploitation."

In most states, when an APS worker suspects a crime has occurred, they will contact local law enforcement and coordinate and/or assist law enforcement on an investigation. APS has a code of ethics that guides their decision making called the National Association of Protected Persons Code of Ethics:

- Adult Protective Services programs and staff promote safety, independence, and quality-of-life for older persons and persons with disabilities who are being mistreated or in danger of being mistreated, and who are unable to protect themselves.
- Every action taken by Adult Protective Services must balance the duty to protect the safety of the vulnerable adult with the adult's right to self-determination.
- Adults have the right to be safe.
- Adults retain all their civil and constitutional rights, i.e., the right to live their lives as they wish, manage their own finances, enter into contracts, marry, etc. unless a court adjudicates otherwise.
- Adults have the right to make decisions that do not conform with societal norms as long as these decisions do not harm others.
- Adults have the right to accept or refuse services. [10]

You may begin to notice a trend here. The concept that people have the right to fail certainly sounds understandable. Dr. Allen S. Teel is a long-time advocate of aging while living in community and the dignity of risk for elders. He formed Full Circle America, a turnkey enterprise started in Maine that "supports elders living in the comfort of their own homes, living their lives to the fullest using technology, social networking, life management, and expansive volunteering." [11] He states in his book *Alone and Invisible No More: How Grassroots Community Action and 21st Century Technologies Can Empower Elders and Stay in the Homes and Lead Healthier, Happier Lives* that to him "the dignity of risk (means) we do not have the option of saying we will only embrace a course of action if it is guaranteed to succeed . . . this time of life requires making the best choice with the information you have at hand and moving forward." [12]

However, when it is your family member who is clearly at risk for self-harm, you may feel less inclined to consider their rights. Some families make the decision to seek guardianship, which is predicated on evidence suggesting that a person does not have the capacity to make decisions in their own self-interest. Capacity generally means the "ability to understand the nature and effects of one's actions."[13]

> Among older adults who are vulnerable to self-neglect, the capacity to make decisions may remain intact. However, the capacity to identify and extract oneself from harmful situations, circumstances, or relationships may be diminished. A key ethical and clinical branch point in identifying older adults at risk for self-neglect involves determining whether the individual can both make and implement decisions regarding personal needs, health, and safety.[14]

It is beyond the scope of this book to get into a detailed conversation about guardianship. However, it is a recourse that has the potential to be sought out by more and more families as a way of hopefully gaining control over a deteriorating healthcare and/or financial situation and overcoming resistance. People are living longer, and dementia is on the rise. There is a massive transfer of wealth from a World War II generation to baby boomers. Families can look to guardianship as a way to prevent the wasting of an elder's estate and/or making the necessary changes to ensure a safe environment.

What is a guardian? A guardian is "a person, institution, or agency appointed by a court to manage the affairs of certain individuals. The guardian may be given the authority to manage personal and/or financial matters. Each state has specific laws, which govern guardianship proceedings and the guardian activities."[15] Sounds like a nifty solution, doesn't it? As a family guardian you can now hire a private caregiver to come to the home and provide the duties and supports that are so desperately needed. But one thing remains the same. Without cooperation and agreement from your elder, you are only creating an adversarial situation if you force someone to do something they strenuously object to. However, if the situation is truly dire or life threatening, you may need to take action.

Regardless of the capacity of the elder, we recommend a family meeting during which family members bring their concerns and discuss them openly, honestly, and patiently. Acknowledge the concepts of autonomy and independence and your efforts to respect a person's decisions even if you disagree with those decisions. If it seems appropriate, let the person know that should things become too dangerous or risky to ignore, you will take action. If this scenario should occur or even if you convince the senior to accept services through a home care agency or home health agency, the agency may refuse to provide care.

It is important to know that even if you convince someone to accept services, private duty agencies we have talked to say that they will not hesitate to deny services to an individual if the home has hygiene issues or self-neglect necessitates the agency calling Adult Protective Services. If the agency feels their staff cannot perform their duties safely, they will decline to provide those services.

In the realm of privately hired care, the issue of an elder person's questionable judgment versus their safety can be equally vexing. Consider this example: a confident and determined elder with advanced Parkinson's insisted on going up the stairs to her bedroom every night. Her two private caregivers, independent contractors who were not from an agency and did not have professional supervision, could not agree whether they should refuse to help their client with her wish or honor her request by assisting her. This created a further problem that caregivers face personally. By assisting someone who has limited mobility and balance to get up the stairs, they put their own safety at risk. It is possible in that scenario that the client may start to fall, the caregiver could try to stop the fall, and the caregiver could become a human cushion and sustain injuries of their own. All varieties of healthcare professionals in any sort of inpatient and outpatient settings have been injured helping patients. Does the client's right to choose a risky behavior supersede the safety of others?

A medical home health agency (short-term services ordered by a physician and covered by insurance) can also limit the kinds of services it provides and the types of conditions it will cover. If you need services that the home health agency does not provide, the agency can choose to reject you as a patient as long as its policies are consistent for all patients. We know of agencies that will honor their intake nurse's opinion that a situation is too dangerous for their staff to provide services.

In addition, home health agencies can refuse to take someone as a patient if they do not believe that they can ensure the patient's safety. For example, if someone needs 'round-the-clock personal care in addition to services the home health agency provides but is opting to go without that care, the agency could find the situation unsafe and not accept the individual as a patient.[16] When a home health nurse goes to a home to do an initial assessment of an individual, they can refuse to provide services to that person based on their own subjective evaluation. Nurses have told us that some of the reasons they deny services are the following: bugs, other sanitary issues, drug use, fall risk, home safety issues like hoarding or obvious mechanical dangers in the home, and sexual advances, to name a few. Don't assume just because someone agrees to allow help in the home that a company will be willing to provide it.

Honoring someone's wishes while still providing offers of support and respect is a fine and sometimes difficult line to walk. Our conversation with Charlie and his journey with his parents is a good example of that experience.

Charlie's Journey

Charlie has been a long-distance care provider for his parents, Martha and Don, for over ten years. This entailed regular phone calls and periodic visits to assess how they were doing and what help they needed. Charlie lives in a good-sized metropolitan area in the Midwest, while his parents have resided in a small town of just fifteen thousand people in Oregon. Like many older adults their age, they have lived in the same town for decades, made friends, had careers, and raised a family. And like the experience of so many other families, the children matured and left for school and jobs in bigger cities where there was more opportunity.

As Charlie's parents aged, they became more isolated in their home, and as their friends have died off, there increasingly seemed little point to them in going out because there was no one they knew to see and nothing to do. They both began to slow down a bit, but any physical problems that arose they just dealt with. They would tell Charlie, "We don't like doctors. They don't do anything anyway." Don continued to drive even though he has significant vision problems and had banged up the car numerous times. He drove short distances to get groceries. Over time, Martha rarely left the house.

Charlie's visits, which were every three to four months, became more frequent as he noticed Don and Martha's declining physical health. The house that they had lived in for decades was chock full of stuff. There were rugs and other fall risks in the house, and routine maintenance like repairs, painting, and cleaning had not been done in years. Charlie broached the topic of getting some assistance in the home: cleaning, mowing the lawn, cooking, and personal care. Both Don and Martha were adamant that they were "doing just fine." They absolutely did not want anyone coming into the home. Charlie's sister, who had not been actively involved in Don and Martha's care, began to pressure Charlie to "do something immediately," insisting that their parents were in danger, the house was a mess, and they were isolated and lonely and needed to be moved as soon as possible.

Charlie increased his visits, although the travel distance made it difficult. As Don and Martha began to have more serious problems, he talked to them both about moving and relocating to the town where he lived into an assisted living facility. Again, he met resistance. Then, after a fall landed him in the emergency room, Don was diagnosed with bladder cancer. He underwent radiation treatment, which bought him about six months before the cancer returned and had spread. Don died shortly afterward. Martha declared to her son: "I will never go through that."

At this point, Charlie implored his mother to move near him. She said she would consider it but then said that she was happy in her own home and did not want to move. Charlie's sister ramped up her pressure for Charlie to force Martha to leave, which he stated he would not do.

Instead he visited his mother more frequently, and after Martha had gone to bed he quietly did home repairs, like replacing light bulbs with LEDs that wouldn't burn out as frequently, installed grab bars in the bathroom, fixed the stair railings, changed out dangerous light switches, and fixed doors. When something major needed repair in the home and Charlie wasn't there, he had a list of contractors he called to do repairs. Martha would allow someone to come in for major work at the home. During the day, Charlie and his mother went out occasionally to eat at a restaurant or go to the cemetery. They began to have conversations about his mother's life and grew closer.

Then Martha began to get weaker. Charlie talked her into going to the doctor, who misdiagnosed her with a heart problem. At this point Martha agreed to home health coming in three times a week. She didn't improve. Weeks later she too ended up in the emergency room and was diagnosed with stage 4 lung cancer, confirming her worst fears about doctors. Two and a half weeks later she died after being sent to a skilled nursing home.

Charlie says this about the decisions he made while caring for his parents long distance: "I believed in respecting my parents' wishes to remain in their home. You have to ask yourself: what is the goal? If the goal is to make things easier on myself, then that is not honoring my parents' wishes. It is not about me or my feelings, it is about them. I was not willing to risk compromising my relationship with my parents to make them safe. I believe in negotiation and cooperative planning to try and reach a consensus. People need to be intrinsically motivated to do something, not extrinsically motivated. If my parents did something just because I wanted it, they would never be happy and I knew that."

You and your family will make decisions about where your elder family members live and how they live in their last years. Those decisions will sometimes be fraught with disagreement, doubt, and ambivalence about whether the chosen path is right or wrong. When a caregiver is involved, you are bringing in the beliefs and rights of another person who may agree or disagree with your elder's wishes for autonomy. It is a complex world of aging that we live in, but one that will present a vast new arena of debate about our rights as human beings throughout our lifespan.

TAKEAWAY POINTS FOR THIS CHAPTER

- Understanding the elder individual's history, upbringing, and culture can bring their personal life view of independence into focus.
- The medicalization of aging has created an unrealistic expectation that medical science can improve quality of life in older age. While clearly life expectancy has been extended, at present there is much evidence that the likelihood of disability also increases in old age.
- Adult children of elders often want to find a quick fix to their parents' need for care. However, if possible, slow down and consider your parent as adults first and people with all the rights that being an adult implies.
- Elders are increasingly vocal about maintaining their autonomy and control. Consider their point of view and their rights to make decisions about their own health care and lifestyle.
- The dignity of risk is a concept that is taking hold with many seniors and their families. It is likely to continue to cause contention with families who have any members whose priority is absolute safety above individual rights.
- Guardianship is an option for families that believe they have no other choice in order to protect their elder family member.

7

THE CAREGIVER RELATIONSHIP

Friendship, Balance, and Boundaries

INTRODUCTION

Having a hired caregiver assisting an elder in the elder's home is a unique situation. Not only does the home become a healthcare setting, it becomes a place of employment and a workplace. There are two very important human beings involved. One is the client who is an older person usually struggling to understand and accept how differently he or she is able or not able to control daily life. The other person in this equation is a caregiver. The caregiver, whom you have carefully hired, usually comes with empathy for the senior's situation and training on how to successfully assist a person in need. That person may or may not have a similar point of view to the individual needing help. The two individuals may have a lot in common or nothing in common other than being together for what can be many hours of the day. Over time, the two people in this honored partnership may find that their knowledge and understanding of each other moves beyond a working relationship. A friendship may form and in many cases they may begin to feel like part of each other's family.

Some sandwich generation family members may liken the experience of hiring and having a caregiver for an elder to hiring a nanny. In both situations, you must interview many applicants until you find someone with whom you feel comfortable, and you must do background checks to ensure that the person you are considering is going to be safe with your child or elder as well as maintaining the safety of your home. Both a nanny and a caregiver make sure that the stove is turned off, the doors are locked, and the faucet is not left on. You are usually looking for someone who has experience and who seems to enjoy being with that particular age group. The real difference is the skill set that you are looking for in a professional caregiver. Many good babysitters and nannies have no more training than a CPR certificate. Their experience with children, often with their own siblings or children, is what is most important. The skills needed to assist an elder at home are quite different. They involve health and safety in more complex ways than most children need. And as we discussed in the last chapter, dealing with the rights of an adult are worlds apart from dealing with those of children. It takes a person who has an appreciation of the elder as an adult.

The elder and caregiver have a dynamic relationship that can have shifting priorities. The elder is the resident of the home and the client. His or her role is both one of control, in that they are the employer, and of vulnerability, because they need another person's help. On the other hand, the caregiver too has a somewhat conflicting combination of roles. First, they are a hired professional employee with a specific job description that entails the completion of daily tasks centered on the client's needs. At the same time, they are physically stronger and sometimes better able to communicate than their client. The caregiver may also be required by an agency or family members to follow through with activities that the elder may not want. The caregiver must weigh such decisions about care with professionalism and respect.

Some people are more comfortable in the position of being in charge on either side of the equation. A senior might be very used to wielding whatever control they have over other people (picture the retired type A executive), and conversely, a caregiver may be very dedicated to getting things done in a timely manner that may or may not suit the elder. Yet again, the senior may be meek and acquiesce to the directives of a caregiver, or you may have a caregiver who is intimidated by a demanding elder. In a better scenario, the two can share the power: one can make concessions to the other to get tasks done and vice versa. It is a balance that those two parties alone will have to work out. No matter how many other concerned players try to intervene (the daughter, the agency supervisor, the doctor, the wife), these two people will need to work cooperatively together. In the process a strong bond can form. If it doesn't, it may be a strained relationship that will not last very long.

We have suggested in past chapters that even though you may be apprehensive about how well you or your family member might get along with this new person in your life, you may also be pleasantly surprised. Much like in any work setting, when two people set out to solve a problem together, they share a common experience and it is usually a positive one. Of course, it doesn't always happen with the first person who walks in the door. A good, intuitive caregiver will adapt to the situation no matter how challenging it may be.

For example, sometimes dementia will cause the elder to be confused about who the caregiver is. Mary had been working with her client Celeste during the day hours for about a month when she was asked to do an overnight shift. In the middle of the night, Celeste got out of bed and, on seeing Mary in her home, demanded to know who she was. Mary tried to explain that they knew each other, but this made Celeste even more agitated and upset. She insisted that Mary leave the house immediately. Mary did not know what to do. She went outside and Celeste quickly locked the door behind her. Mary knocked on the door and Celeste opened it briefly and yelled at Mary, "I thought I told you to get out of here!" It was 3 a.m. and cold outside and Mary went to her car parked in front of the house. She had left her cell phone in the house. Now what would she do? A little bit later, she noticed Celeste standing in front of the window in her house. Celeste saw Mary in the car and waved at her. Mary waved back. Celeste waved her arm indicating Mary should come to the door. Mary walked up to the door and Celeste opened it and said, "What are you doing out there in the cold? Come inside!"

Most of us have experienced getting personal care to our physical body in a doctor's office, a hospital, a dentist's office, a hair salon, or a massage studio. Having personal care with someone who is not a member of your family physically touching you, lifting you, bathing you, and dressing you in your own home is a very different matter. In some cases, the elder suffers a great deal of anxiety about this, and sometimes it is their adult children who are more apprehensive.

A caregiver, Sonia, tells the story of a ninety-one-year-old client. Her only task was to prepare food for him. She microwaved food and pureed it because he had difficulty swallowing. One day he complained of difficulty breathing and he went to the hospital. He came back after a couple of days and he needed a shower. The family asked Sonia if she could give her client a shower, because that was normally not part of her assigned tasks, and she said yes. "I have showered many people. I got him ready to get him into the shower, and he said 'aren't you getting in with me?' And I said no, but after that he thought I was his girlfriend! And this was after going in to help him for months. He was so happy that I was going to be his girlfriend. He told me 'I have money.' I told him I had a boyfriend. He was just so lonely and wanted companionship."

MAYBE IT WOULD BE EASIER TO HIRE A FAMILY MEMBER? PLANNING IS KEY

While the focus of this book is on hiring nonfamily caregivers, many families do find that a paid family care provider is a good solution. We are glad to see a trend in states that have either grants or Medicaid funding to pay some family caregivers to care for their elder family members. Many family caregivers are overworked, overstressed, and never paid for their labor. About 34 million Americans provided unpaid care to an adult age fifty or older in 2015, according to the National Alliance for Caregiving and AARP.[1] Some states and local area boards of aging are trying to compensate family caregivers. There is an excellent online tool on the website payingforseniorcare.com (https://www .payingforseniorcare.com/paid-caregiver/program-locator.html) to help you find out if you are eligible as a family member to be paid to provide care for a senior family member. Or you can call your local area board of aging and find out if this would be a possibility for your family.

Experts in this area agree that much of the same planning we advise for hiring someone outside of family should occur.[2] Just as in any work setting, it is important to communicate the tasks of the job and maintain supervision. That means having family meetings with all parties present to discuss and agree on what care needs to be provided, when and where that care will occur, how many hours the family caregiver is expected to work in a week, how coverage will be provided when that person is absent or on vacation, and what will be fair compensation. A work agreement that includes these points should be in writing and the family caregiver and the employer (the elder or their power of attorney) should sign it.[3]

Families should follow these steps to avoid misunderstanding about the job and to keep family discord at minimum. One caregiver we know, Annette, had been working full time as a private hire caregiver. After work, she would go home to take care of her elderly Aunt Estelle, whom she lived with as unpaid home care. It was very stressful and exhausting, especially when she would need to get up several times in the middle of the night to help her aunt to the bathroom and then have to get up later to go to her regular job. Finally, she and Estelle learned that a family member could be paid to be Estelle's caregiver for a certain number of hours per week through a local county grant. Estelle picked her youngest daughter Sylvia to be the paid family caregiver. Annette was thrilled that she would get a break and she moved to her own place. However, when she would come to visit her aunt, she discovered that Sylvia had not been there at the designated hours; Estelle had not been bathed or been dressed in clean clothes. Annette was in a very difficult position: Should she tell the county liaison that her cousin was not doing her job? Would her aunt be angry at her for blowing the whistle? She did not know what to do. Fortunately, the county supervisor found out on her own, ended the grant for the daughter's service, and eventually worked it out for Annette to get the position. Though it paid much less than Annette's private hire salary, she was very happy to do it.

FAMILY CONFIDENTIAL: HOW PRIVACY MATTERS TO YOU AND YOUR FAMILY

Every family has a particular way that they treat their privacy. For some, it is a family mandate that bodily functions are not to be discussed or displayed in or out of the family. Think about what your parents told you never to mention in public. These topics can run the gamut: don't talk about personal finances, a family member's illness, your sister's bad math grades, or what your father really thinks of the next door neighbor. Or you may remember being on the way to a larger family gathering, such as for Thanksgiving, when mom turned to the kids in the back seat and said, "And remember, no one is to ask where Uncle George is. You know Grandma doesn't like to be reminded that he left Aunt Susie."

Privacy is not always a matter of secrecy, but rather, as defined by the Merriam-Webster Dictionary, it is "the state of being apart from others."[4]

We need our privacy in a world of "too much information." With privacy, we are not necessarily hiding negative conditions or knowledge, but rather we have comfort in having something personal that we only share with our immediate tribe.

After hiring a caregiver, it can be difficult to know what to expect in terms of confidentiality and professional, appropriate behavior. Caregivers themselves are often at a loss if they haven't had adequate training about what is expected when working in someone's home environment. Others are well aware of agency confidentiality policies, but violate those policies knowingly. Ask the agency you are hiring for a copy of those policies. Much of what is expected of caregivers is not necessarily offered during any kind of formal training and this leaves workers to fend for themselves in making day-to-day decisions about what is appropriate.

As this partnership develops, there can be some rocky moments as caregiver and elder do the delicate dance of acknowledging what is acceptable and what is not. For example, some people are very uncomfortable with "bathroom talk" and consider this not only a breach of privacy, but simply not appropriate or classy. Loss of independence doesn't have to mean loss of privacy or respect. Here are some examples of how both client and caregiver can communicate and set boundaries for privacy.

- Don is a World War II veteran who, despite being confined to a wheelchair, has tremendous pride in his service and his independence. His new caregiver starts her relationship by saying: "Honey, it is so nice to meet you." Don responds by saying: "I am only one person's honey and that is my deceased wife's." Point taken.
- Cecile has continence problems along with difficulty walking due to a hip replacement. Her new caregiver, Lynn, is hired to assist her with some cooking, cleaning, and getting to the bathroom. Lynn is a seasoned caregiver and begins the relationship by asking how Cecile would like to be approached when dealing with bathroom issues. She asks questions like: Do you prefer that I go in the bathroom with you? Should I just stay outside the door and when you are ready you can let me know? If there are other people around how would you like to handle the situation if you need help going to the bathroom?
- In contrast, it can be a challenge for a caregiver to maintain his or her own privacy. One day, Lorraine was at her longtime client's

home. She had excused herself to use the restroom. She had on a pair of nice dress slacks with a side zipper. As she reached to pull up her pant zipper, the whole zipper ripped out into her hand. She had no zipper and her pants were flapping open. She pulled her long sweater down as far as she could and went out meekly to her client and said, "Do you by any chance have any safety pins?" Her client asked why and Lorraine told her. Her client said, "Well show me, I'm pretty good at fixing these things." "I told her that I was too embarrassed for her to see my undergarments! And my client said to me, 'Why should you? You see mine all the time!' So I let her help me with the safety pins and she was pretty proud of the job she did and that she helped me out."

- A new caregiver was helping an elderly client who was in great pain whenever she was transferred from her bed to her chair. In fact, the elder woman usually let out a string of curse words at this time that would make a sailor proud. The caregiver, who was very religious, was appalled and actually said to the client's niece, "I always find that it's the ones that haven't been saved that have the greatest pain and suffering." The niece kept her anger below the surface and told the caregiver that in fact, her aunt was a good and honorable person and that her religion was her private business. The niece discussed the incident with the supervisor and made it clear that if this type of judgment occurred again or had any negative effect on her aunt's care, she would go to another agency.

We have talked about the fact that the desire to stay in one's home is the preference of most elders, but with that decision comes a loss of privacy that many people do not anticipate. Privacy is expressed through conversation, behavior, and attitude from both elder and caregiver. And although we are focused on the privacy of the elder, caregivers also deserve and often desire to keep their personal lives confidential.

Let's take a look at some of the basic areas of importance to a caregiving situation with regard to privacy and confidentiality.

HIPAA and Confidentiality

As a consumer you may have heard of HIPAA. When you go to a doctor's office you may be required to sign a document stating that you understand the confidentiality requirements of the physician's office. Trying to get medical information about your elder or other family member can be a nightmare without signed releases or healthcare power of attorney due to HIPAA regulations.

HIPAA is the Health Insurance and Portability and Accountability Act. It is legislation that provides data privacy and security provisions for safeguarding medical information. This is an enormously complex act and misunderstood by many healthcare providers. The intent would seem very reasonable on the face of it: to protect your healthcare information and require your permission to release that information. However, families caring for an ailing elder have experienced firsthand the enormous frustration of trying to coordinate multiple healthcare entities to share information vital to someone's care.

The question is: Is a privately hired caregiver bound by HIPAA regulations and does it matter? According to the World Privacy Forum, "A simple rule of thumb is that any provider who bills an insurance company or health plan is a covered entity under HIPAA. If your doctor accepts Medicare, for example, the doctor is a covered entity. A free health clinic may not be subject to HIPAA because it doesn't bill anyone. A doctor who charges every patient $25 cash and does not submit a bill to any insurance company may not be covered by HIPAA. A first aid room at your workplace may or may not be covered by HIPAA. If you want to know if the organization you are dealing with is a HIPAA covered entity, ask. If you don't get a straight answer, ask for a copy of its privacy policy. If it has a privacy policy, the policy will explain about HIPAA's application. If it doesn't have a written privacy policy, then it is either not covered by HIPAA or it is violating the rule."[5]

Under this definition, private duty agencies are not bound by HIPAA because they do not bill insurance. In our experience, however, most reputable agencies abide by the intent of this law in training their staff not to share confidential information without the client's consent. If you are hiring privately or through an online company, it falls on you to explain what your wishes are with regard to privacy. You may be asking yourself under what conditions this may be important. Here are some examples:

- Simone is incontinent and has to make certain that she has protection when she goes into the community. She has a caregiver at home to assist her with everyday tasks like housekeeping and cooking. A friend comes to the house to take Simone to church, and the caregiver says, "Simone will be ready in a minute. She has to change her Depends." Well, Simone's friend does not know that Simone has incontinence problems. Simone has wanted to keep this private because she is ashamed of the fact she has to manage this problem.

- Jeffrey lives alone in his own home with substantial help from daily caregivers. Jeffrey has been diagnosed with Alzheimer's disease, but he is still a spunky, social person who enjoys going to the senior center twice a week with his caregiver. He is able to play a simple card game called 'Uno" with some other men he has met at the center. During one of these games, he completely loses track of how to play the game when his turn comes. The caregiver says, "Oh, Jeffrey has Alzheimer's so his memory isn't good." Most likely Jeffrey's senior center friends noticed that he was slower and had memory problems, but to hear the term Alzheimer's has a diminishing effect on their view of Jeffrey.

Bottom line: any older adult's physical or mental health information should be kept private unless permission is given by the person or a family member who deems this information important for healthcare purposes. To ensure that confidentiality is protected, we recommend leaving nothing to chance. Speak with the caregiver(s) yourself and be clear and firm in the following:

1. Under no circumstances is medical or mental health information to be provided to anyone other than designated healthcare professionals, and even then only when permission is given by the client.
2. If the elder is capable of providing exceptions to this expectation, then it is their right to allow the caregiver to share information that they agree is permissible.
3. Some healthcare entities stringently abide by HIPAA, making it difficult for a caregiver who may accompany an elder to a physician's office to share or obtain information. Be prepared for this circumstance by allowing the caregiver and client to sign a release of information at the physician's office.

THE INTERVIEW: STARTING THE RELATIONSHIP OFF RIGHT AT THE BEGINNING

With some differences between a private hire and hiring with an agency, you will have an opportunity to meet and interview the caregiver. With an agency, approach this with flexibility. It is more unusual to interview individual caregivers when hiring through a care agency, but you can request it. Some agencies have told us that it is rare for families to ask for an interview with specific caregivers after they have interviewed the supervisor and administrative staff of the agency. They do not encourage it as it is more costly for them administratively and working caregivers are not always available to come in for short periods of time for additional interviewing. One supervisor shared that in the instances that she has arranged this at a client's request, it was awkwardly more like a beauty contest than an actual interview. The client was more interested in literally looking the person over than delving into their work history. Another supervisor handles this in a different way so that the elder never has a total stranger show up alone to work with them. The supervisor always comes with a new caregiver to the new client's home to introduce them in a "meet and greet," goes over all of the caregiving tasks with the family and caregiver present, has the elder and family show them where things are, and then leaves them together. In the case of an established client, she will always have a supervisor or a known caregiver there to introduce and orient a new caregiver so that there is always a responsible handoff of care.

If you have interviewed different care agencies before settling on one, you will have asked them very specific questions about their hiring and interviewing process: What kinds of questions do you ask potential employees? What types of experience and certification do you seek in a candidate? What is your background check and drug screening process like? You and your elder should meet with the agency supervisor before getting started and discuss your preference for care and who your ideal caregiver is. More often, you may not be given the benefit of an interview and they will suggest and send a caregiver who they think will be a good fit rather than you having a separate interview. At that time, you can meet and assess how the caregiver does in the home setting, which can have its advantages. Consider this a working interview. How does the caregiver greet and initially settle in with you or your elder? Do they politely ask permission and ask how you want breakfast to be arranged and prepared? Or do they just start rummaging around to find what they think is breakfast? How are they communicating their questions to you and your family? Or are they making assumptions?

If you are hiring privately, you will want to assemble your list of questions for the applicant (see Sample Interview Questions to follow). If you are hiring through an online company, you will be able to read detail about the caregiver's experience and work history and some may have a short interview video that you can watch. Be prepared for the in-person interview to observe cues and behaviors that can tell you a lot about the person you are considering hiring. For example:

- Is the person on time for the interview?
- When asked about previous employment, does the caregiver say negative things about the agency or clients?
- Does the caregiver share specific personal information, such as names and medical history of previous clients?
- Does the person have other jobs and obligations that may interfere with the schedule of care that you need?
- How does the caregiver talk about old people? One agency supervisor advises, "Listen for the person who tells you how much they care about an older person in their life or a previous client. That tells you a lot about how they view the people that they are helping."
- Does the person become nervous or bristle at the prospect of having a background check or drug screening? This should be par for the course for experienced caregivers and something that they do willingly as it improves the reliability of their profession.

Sample Interview Questions:[6]

1. Tell me a little about yourself and what interests you in this job?
2. What experience do you have working with elders? Do you have any certification such as a Certified Nurse Assistant (CNA) or training for CPR?
3. My family member has (Parkinson's, dementia, problems with balance, etc.). The care involves these responsibilities and tasks (be sure to include a discussion of any lifting needed). Do you have experience with people who have had these conditions?

4. Tell me how you would handle a problem that arises. For example, my mother has dementia. What would you do if she became upset because she thought she needed to leave the house for an appointment that she doesn't actually have?

5. Here are the hours that we need. Are you available these hours and for this schedule? Are you available for other times that may come up? How far is your commute to this residence? Tell me about other jobs or obligations that you have outside of this one.

6. Do you smoke? Even some good caregivers are embarrassed to admit that they smoke. It is a good opportunity to clarify your expectations. Designate an outdoor smoking area and make it clear that this is the only place smoking is allowed.

7. Do you drive and do you have a clean driving record? Would you be comfortable driving your own vehicle or my family's car? Does your car have insurance? (If you prefer to have the caregiver drive your family's vehicle, check with your insurance company to make sure you have given them the information that they need.)

8. Explain that you require a background check and drug screening as well as at least two references from previous work. Some very good information can come up at this juncture. If someone tells you up front that they have something on their record related to a domestic abuse situation in which all parties were cited as some jurisdictions have done, and you can verify that there are no other violations, you have a choice to make a judgment that this person was not a perpetrator but a victim and is still a good candidate for the job. If the caregiver is very young with limited work experience, the reference may be a teacher, a pastor, or some other non-family member.

9. Discuss that you will have a simple employment contract.

10. Go over all the employment details:

- Discuss salary and payroll taxes. What has your previous hourly wage been at your last job?
- Discuss how you will handle vacation hours and coverage when sick.
- Collect name, address, phone numbers, and e-mail addresses. You don't want a great caregiver to walk out of the house and you don't have their full contact info.

- Ask for an emergency contact.
- Have the candidates that you wish to hire sign a permission form to run a background check (available through the company that you use to do the check or you can use an online company's form as a template).
- Have W-4 tax forms and your employment agreement at the ready if there is a great candidate that you want to hire on the spot.
- Explain that there will be a probation or grace period if you, the elder, or the caregiver find that it is not a good fit. Let them know how frequently performance will be evaluated.

If you are of a certain age and you have not been involved in an interviewing situation for a while, you may be aghast at some of the behaviors, expectations, and remarks that have become sadly commonplace in interviews and employment settings these days. First, people don't show up for the interview. They don't call to tell you that, they simply do not show up. People you do hire don't show up for their first shift and never give you the courtesy of telling you. In fact, one care agency supervisor told us that she has had great caregivers who have, in some instances, worked with one client for two years and then suddenly don't show up for their Saturday day shift and are never heard from again.

The supervisors and hiring staff at care agencies can tell you all about strange interviews and applicants. One told us that she has had a caregiver applicant bring her mother and her baby into the interview room. She also had scarily long fingernails that the supervisor couldn't help but envision digging into the fragile skin of her elder clients. Another applicant brought her husband in for the interview too. And there was the applicant who had such bad personal hygiene that after she left, the staff had to air out the chair outside that the applicant had sat in. One applicant, after having gone for her drug screening but before the employer got the results back, called to talk about it. She explained that the agency shouldn't worry about that cocaine that was going to show up on her screening. "Really, I have never done it before, it was just a one-time thing. A friend came over the other night and suggested that I might like to try it, so I thought, okay, why not! But, it just gave me a headache, so I won't be doing that again, alright?"

We don't tell you these stories to frighten you but to forewarn you that interviewing can be tricky. As one supervisor related, for every twenty applicants that are not appropriate to be caregivers, there is one person who stands out among the rest and has the qualities and skills that you are looking for, whom you can relate to with trust and good feelings. The available caregiver pool has always had the potential to be "feast or famine." It can seem like just when you are in need of a good caregiver, there are none to be found. There can be a seasonal element to your search, as many nursing students work part time as caregivers and their school schedules may change their availability. The traditional career caregivers may have already found long-term caregiving jobs and tend to stay in them for the duration. Without them in the mix, there are simply a lot of people who do not have "the calling" to be the best caregivers. However, it is a reality of caring for the elderly that over time, people pass away or possibly move on to a facility. Then the desirable caregivers are back in our midst and available again. Timing is everything in your search!

WHAT COULD POSSIBLY GO WRONG?

Even with good intentions, some caregiver situations take a turn for the worse. It can be a simple miscommunication that delays important care interventions from happening. For example, suppose a doctor calls the son after office hours to tell him that his mother's labs came back and she needs to increase her fluid intake. The son is about to get on a flight for a business conference that will have him tied up for the entire next day. Even though he calls the agency and the on-call person tells him that she will convey the doctor's instructions to the caregiver in the morning, there are times when the message can get delayed or even misunderstood.

In addition to pitfalls with communication, there is the very real problem of downtime in a caregiving setting and some caregivers not having enough supervision or self-motivation to make the best use of it. Though some states have nursing home standards of care requiring two to three hours of hands-on care per resident per day, the real number generally falls below that.[7] In a home care setting there are more tasks for an individual caregiver to attend to. After all, they do the meal preparation and the cleaning, laundry, and transportation and other tasks that in a facility would be the job of another person. But once a routine is established to do meals and personal care such as bathing and dressing, there can be quite a bit of unstructured time. Depending on the skills and motivation of the caregiver, the amount of supervision, and the engagement with the client, some caregivers may choose to take a break most of that time. A good-quality caregiver will use that time to take the client on outings and visits with friends or community resources, or if the client is homebound to find some sort of home activities to stimulate thinking and memory. A not so good caregiver will not use that time in the service of the client's needs.

This really is more important than you think and can have unfavorable consequences for the elder. For example, one elder we know had foot surgery and was sent home with her caregiver, but was unable to get up on her foot and do things from her normal routine. The agency sent different caregivers on different days. On the days one caregiver came, the day was full of morning routines, the caregiver helping the elder call friends and family, coloring and drawing, doing exercises that the physical therapist had recommended, and going outside in the wheelchair for a bit of fresh air. The caregiver was action oriented. That day, the elder complained little of pain except for "I'm a little uncomfortable, but I'm fine." The next day, a different caregiver came. After the perfunctory morning care was done, the client was parked in front of the TV for the rest of day except for meals. The caregiver spent most of her time on her phone checking her Facebook feed, speaking to the client only when necessary. On that day, the elder experienced more pain, was more restless during the night, and needed to have a narcotic to quell the pain.

Even though the first caregiver/client day in the example above may seem comparatively like a quiet day for a younger person, having small but diverse items on the agenda for the day makes a huge difference for someone with less daily activity. Variety and mental stimulation take many forms for the elderly. A caregiver who is thinking of their client as whole person will anticipate that with careful planning and an appropriate level of activity. You and your elder family member should discuss with the agency or the private hire caregiver what your expectations are for a typical day, even for a day when the client has low energy. What do you expect them to do at a minimum?

BOUNDARIES: GOOD FENCES MAKE GOOD NEIGHBORS

Having a proactive, involved caregiver can be a dream come true. But sometimes the very attributes that make for a good caregiver can cross professional lines, and boundaries become blurred. We have seen situations in which a caregiver is so assertive and involved that they begin to make decisions on behalf of the elder they are caring for. Or, they become too much of an influence on the elder.

Caregivers can be amazingly astute and intuitive about the person they are caring for. This is a good thing. However, it is important that the relationship remain professional. Here are some reasons why:

- As we have shown, elders can be more easily influenced by someone they like and care about. They can subvert their own wants and needs in the service of someone they feel close to.
- Caregivers can absolutely be friendly, but not friends. One unfortunate consequence of a close relationship is when the caregiver leaves their employment. This can have a profound effect on an elder who has grown very close to a caregiver and can happen regardless of the nature of their relationship.
- Professional boundaries encourage good decision making. A good dose of objectivity helps a caregiver make the best decisions on behalf of the person they are caring for. Alice is an eighty-three-year-old woman with diabetes. Her physician has recommended a diabetic diet that restricts the sweets that Alice loves so much. Her caregiver, Danielle, has been working with Alice for over a year and they get along great. Danielle has become so close to Alice that she is often referred to by Alice as "my other daughter." Danielle has been very careful to gently correct Alice by saying, "That is a wonderful compliment, but you have your family and I am here to support and care for you." Alice continually but politely pushes Danielle to be lenient regarding her dietary restrictions, pleading, "Just one piece of chocolate today!" Danielle knows that she must not give in to these requests, but it is very hard to say no and she worries when Alice gets angry. Danielle doesn't want to negatively affect their good relationship. Danielle explains that she has to abide by the instructions on the plan of care provided by her office and she has no control to change decisions that have been made by

Alice's healthcare providers, but she adds, "I know what it is like to have to deny yourself something that gives you such pleasure. I have to watch my salt intake because of high blood pressure, and I love salt!"

BRINGING FAMILY MEMBERS OR PETS TO AN ELDER'S HOME

Believe it or not, this happens more than you might think. As a care provider becomes comfortable with the person they are taking care of, a relationship is formed. Intimate tasks are often part of the caregiving experience, and even when they aren't, caregiver and client grow close. This can be a very positive experience but, as we have seen in chapter 5, can lead to exploitation if the caregiver is unscrupulous. It can also encourage unprofessional behavior.

We have observed countless situations in which a caregiver brings children, pets, babies, siblings, and other relatives to an elder's home during their shift. There may be a more understandable reason caregivers bring babies, toddlers, and other young people to someone's house. Many of these workers have to arrange child care or have other challenging situations that necessitate (in their eyes) bringing a child to someone's home when their child care arrangements fall through. In some cases the care provider may bring a pet or baby to an elder's home thinking that this would be a positive experience for the elder.

Caregivers with visiting pets can be greatly beneficial to some elders if permission is asked and it is understood that it is strictly the choice of the elder and family. In fact, some care agencies have "therapy dogs" that may visit their clients. Some agencies connect pet-owning caregivers with pet-loving clients. Some private hire caregivers ask permission to bring their pets (usually small dogs) with them to work once or twice a week. As always, the most important variable here is that it is the choice of the elder and that they give permission. Of the many losses that elders face, losing a pet is one of the saddest. Being a lifetime responsible pet owner and realizing that a new pet will likely outlive them leads most elders (or their families) to the conclusion that they can no longer be pet owners. However, the amazing bond between humans and pets does not disappear as one ages. In fact, that unconditional love that we receive and give with our cats and dogs greatly enhances our sense of well-being through physical decline and until the end of our lives.

We have also seen situations in which a care provider brings a family member to an elder's home completely convinced that this relative can assist in the assigned duties of care, which in their mind is a good thing! It's also quite possible, when asked their permission first, that a family and elder would welcome a one-time visit or two from the caregiver's family. The key here is to get prior permission and to define the visit as a social one. Beware of any caregiver who suggests that a family member or friend could do work around the home and be paid out of pocket. It may sound convenient, but it is quite likely to cause problems, such as misunderstandings and possible exploitation.

The problem with bringing someone else to a caregiving situation is the liability it creates for the caregiver and the agency or homeowner. A licensed and bonded agency has insurance to cover an employee should something happen to them on the job. Their insurance does not cover anyone else that is not an employee. This opens up the agency and the employee to lawsuit. If this is a private hire situation, the client may incur unwanted liability if there is an injury in the client's home.

FACEBOOK AND OTHER STICKY INTERNET TEMPTATIONS

Social media is a part of our everyday existence, yet many people, especially younger folks, don't really think much about what the privacy implications are. They are so used to posting personal information on the web that it doesn't really register that what they put out there is available for anyone to see. Boundaries are broken all too often.

Caregivers may blithely enter information under their demographic data that involves your family that you would not want as public information. For instance, caregivers have posted on their social media profile "Work: At the Gerald Smith residence 2015–Current." They see this as similar to posting "Work: University Hospital 2014–Current." But while that is their workplace, your family and their residence are not a public entity.

Very innocently, some caregivers have said, "Nobody sees it but my friends. Isn't it okay if my friends know that I work here?" So many people, not just caregivers, have no idea about their privacy settings and that if they are not set correctly anyone on their social media site could easily read every post and look at every photo they have on their page. In fact, some people may find this is a very useful tool for assessing potential caregivers in the hiring process.

Another issue that may come up for families and caregivers is when a caregiver asks to friend you on Facebook or connect on another social media site. Of course, you develop a closeness with a person who has such an important role for your family. You may be a person who friends everyone from your first-grade teacher whom you have not seen in decades to your broker and everyone in between. You may use your social media mostly for business purposes or to share family updates with distant relatives. In any case, be aware and make a considered decision about connecting with a caregiver on these sites. It may be best to have a policy that you simply don't do it.

As in so many areas of life, it helps to have an agreement up front defining what the rules are. If you hire through an agency, they have an employee contract that you can ask to see. If you are hiring privately, it is a good idea to write up a brief and simple work agreement to cover some of the points we have discussed in this chapter. A sample of a caregiver work agreement appears in table 7.1.[8] Use this as a template and adjust for your own unique situation. Please be sure to consult a payroll company or do some online research for specific current rules regarding sick and vacation leave in your locality.

WHEN THINGS CLICK

When a caregiver and elder "click," it is a thing of beauty. Caregivers can transform an elder's life in meaningful and lasting ways.

- Getting physical: Caregivers can provide added support and reinforcement of physical therapy goals by being trained to do exercises with an elder. At the very least they can offer reminders and encouragement. An example: Maureen is in her nineties and has had the same caregiver, Jean, for over ten years. They have a simple routine that they follow every week. Every day, Maureen strolls with her walker with Jean by her side to the fitness room in her apartment

Table 7.1. Sample Professional Caregiver Employment Agreement

Name of Professional Caregiver

Address

Home Phone Number

Cell Phone Number

Emergency Contact Name and
Number

Care Recipient Name

Employer Name if Different

SALARY
Hourly/Weekly Salary

Hours per Week

To Be Paid Every:

Overtime Rate for over 40 Hours/
Week

Salary and Performance Review Policy

SCHEDULE
Start Date

Probation Period Ends

Daily Hours

Days Off

Number of Sick Days and Vacation
Days: Applicable after what length of
employment _____ mos./yr

TAX WITHHOLDING/ REPORTING

Employee will complete Form I-9 (available at www.uscis.gov/forms) and provide the required documentation verifying employment eligibility within three days of hiring.

Employer will withhold the required Social Security and Medicare taxes from the employee's pay, along with income taxes per the employee's instructions on Form W-4 and all other applicable state taxes. All tax withholdings will be remitted to the state and federal tax agencies on or before the household employment tax deadlines.

Employer will provide employee with Form W-2 (available at www.irs.gov/ Forms-&-Pubs) at the end of the year (by January 31).

Employer will report employee's earnings to the Social Security Administration so that employee receives appropriate retirement benefits.

Check off when forms complete:

Form I-9 _____

Form W-4 _____

Form W-2 _____

SPECIFIC CAREGIVING TASKS

Medications: Prompt or Give	Yes	No
Personal Care: Transfers	Yes	No
Assist with (circle all that apply):	Bathing Dressing Shaving	Toileting Walking/exercise Personal grooming

MEAL PREPARATION

	Plan _____ meals and _____ snacks a day	Prepare _____ per day Help feed

GENERAL DUTIES
(circle all that apply)
Cleaning and Home
Activities of Daily Living and Errands

- Make bed
- Clean dishes and put away, wipe countertops and dust household surfaces
- Clean bathroom sink, bath, and toilet
- Empty trash in bedroom, bathroom, and kitchen
- Secure home when leaving
- Obtain groceries and supplies with client
- Take client to any appointments
- Faith-based visits
- Reading aloud, coloring, reading the paper
- Playing cards or board games

- Clean linens
  Frequency ____
- Wash, dry, fold clothes
- Vacuum/sweep carpets and floors
- Care for pet and plants
- Sweep/shovel/de-ice front steps
- Put groceries away with client
- Take client to senior center or other social gatherings
- Go on walks and get fresh air
- Provide companionship and conversation

CONFIDENTIALITY

Employee understands that any and all private information obtained about the employers, clients, or their dependents during the course of employment, including but not limited to medical, financial, legal, and career, are strictly confidential and may not be disclosed to any third party for any reason.

Social Media Policy

Employee understands that no information about his/her location, plans for the day, or pictures of family members should be shared on any social media network. Employee will also not tell strangers to the family (that is, caregiver's friends) where he or she is spending the day, unless the family has authorized.

GROUNDS FOR TERMINATION

The following are grounds for immediate termination:
- Allowing the safety of the dependent(s) to be compromised
- Inconsistent or nonperformance of agreed-upon job responsibilities
- Concerning issues in background checks
- Dishonesty
- Stealing
- Misuse of family automobile
- Breach of confidentiality clause
- Persistent absenteeism or tardiness
- Unapproved guests
- Smoking or consumption of alcohol while on duty
- Use of an illegal drug
- Overuse of cell phone or computer while on duty
- Negotiating terms of employment with senior directly
- Failing to report any additional monies or gifts given to caregiver by senior
- _____
- _____
- _____

Employer hereby agrees to be fully bound by the terms of this contract.
Employer Signature: _____
Printed Name: _____
Employer Address: _____
Employer Telephone Number: _____
Employer Email: _____
Date: _____

Employee hereby agrees to be fully bound by the terms of this contract.
Employee Signature: _____
Printed Name: _____
Employee Email: _____
Date: _____

Source: Adapted from "Sample Adult and Senior Care Contract," by Julia Quinn-Sczesuil, Care.com, accessed November 11, 2016, https://www.care.com/c/stories/5429/sample-adult-and-senior-care-contract/.

building. There Jean very carefully helps Maureen onto a small stationary bike. Maureen isn't exactly ready to enter a race, but she does her mandatory twelve minutes on the bike because she knows Jean won't let her get away with less.

- Social engagement: Isolation is a serious and sometimes debilitating condition that can affect elders who find themselves confined to home due to medical or cognitive problems. Simply having someone to talk to can be immensely positive and may have curative effects, raising someone's spirits and improving mood. Oftentimes a caregiver can make the difference in encouraging someone to get out to church again or try a senior center. One older couple we know has had a long and happy social life. However, age has taken a lot of mobility away from them, and memory problems make it difficult to keep up with old friends. Their caregiver came one evening to make their dinner. She announced excitedly that her daughter was part of a national TV talent contest and she wondered if the couple would like to watch the show she was on after dinner. Yes, they were intrigued. Each week, they watched the show together with their caregiver as the caregiver's daughter maintained her spot in the competition. In the final week, the daughter won the national competition! The couple shared that joy with the caregiver and they were all proud for the daughter's accomplishment.

- Mind matters: Elders have a lifetime of activities that they enjoy, but illness or dementia can cut those cherished activities short. A creative caregiver can explore other activities that are possible and offer support to learn those activities. Sometimes a simple change of scenery and getting away from the same four walls can be invigorating, such as a drive into the country or some time in the park can be uplifting. Jimmy is a seventy-three-year-old man with dementia who has short-term memory loss and difficulty connecting with people. Two other caregivers have tried to work with him, but his inappropriate language and mild flirting have caused them to quit. A new caregiver, Chelsey, starts to work with Jimmy. She starts by taking time to get to know him. Jimmy's long-term memory is intact so he is able to talk about growing up in Alabama—what his life was like and what he enjoyed. Chelsey finds out that Jimmy loves being outdoors and has an interest in birds. Chelsey finds an aviary and takes Jimmy there to look at birds, then she takes him to the local park to feed the ducks. She also finds out that Jimmy used to fish and although he can't fish now, they find a pond and watch other people fish. Jimmy thanks Chelsey profusely every time they go out, telling her how much he appreciates being able to be outdoors. His inappropriate language and behavior greatly decreases.

TAKEAWAY POINTS FOR THIS CHAPTER

- Both caregiver and elder bring personalities, history, and values to the relationship.
- The caregiver and elder relationship typically work best when it is a partnership.
- Hiring a family member as the caregiver is an option and some states reimburse the family member for caregiving. Be cautious and diligent when hiring a member of the family.
- Confidentiality and privacy matter. If hiring through an agency, find out what their policies are with regard to client information. If hiring privately or online, make yours and your elder's wishes known ahead of time so there are no misunderstandings.
- If you have the opportunity for a "meet and greet," do so. If hiring through an agency, find out what their interview process consists of. If you are doing the hiring, prepare your questions ahead of time.
- Be prepared for caregiver problems. Despite thorough preparation, problems can arise from incompatibility or boundary and privacy issues.
- Investigate agency policies regarding bringing pets, family members, and children to a client's home. If you are hiring privately, be clear in your own mind about what is acceptable.

8

THROWING IN THE TOWEL

INTRODUCTION

There is no doubt that readers of this book who are aging in place with caregivers or helping a elder family member to do so are fully committed to it. After all, the amount of thought and effort to have a successful life at home with caregivers is a huge undertaking. The information and suggestions that we outline in *Aging with Care* are not easy, overnight solutions. It takes dedication and a positive and flexible attitude to make it work.

Even so, there will be some families who will have to conclude that aging and living at home, even with the assistance of a good caregiver, is not a viable option. There are many reasons that can come together and make living at home impossible. Here is an overview of the primary reasons that we see that result in a move from home to an assisted living facility or nursing home. We will discuss each in more detail in this chapter:

- Cost.
- Changes, complications, or worsening of a medical condition. One of the most likely conditions regardless of diagnosis is an increase in immobility.
- The management of caregivers becomes overwhelming.
- The physical environment of the home is no longer adaptable or it is simply too expensive to do so.
- The medical team may express concern that care at home is not adequate.

There are many reasons that can combine and make the prospect of arranging and managing home care untenable. Sometimes the reasons for considering the move away from home are as unique as the person and their life story.

TWO OLD LIFETIME FRIENDS

Second cousins twice removed, Mike and Waldo had known each other their entire lives. Not only were they family, they also attended the same elementary and high schools. Mike, being a few years older, was always the leader. He enrolled at the local college and encouraged Waldo to follow him. They served in the same branch of the military. After that, Mike and Waldo stayed in their hometown even though other family members moved away. After each had married and had children, there were many family gatherings, outings, and even vacations together. It never seemed like being family was the main reason for their close tie. They were simply each other's best friend.

Many years later in their old age, they each became widowers. Mike's son had arranged a caregiver to assist Mike when he developed some beginning signs of dementia following a difficult recovery from a knee replacement surgery. He had some problems with confusion at night and his son, Jackson, decided that it would be wise to have twenty-four-hour care, so a second caregiver was hired for that. Jackson had hired them privately, but decided to have an agency fill the job on the weekends.

Waldo had been living with his daughter Lavonne in her home. Lavonne worked full time and had partial custody of her grandson, who had some learning disabilities. All was working well until Lavonne was laid off from her job. Her job search locally was fruitless, but she heard through a former co-worker in a town a few hours away of a job in her field and she quickly went to apply and to her relief was hired. She had been considering relocating for some time because she was sure that her grandson would do better in a different school system that offered more than the local school. It would even be a better fit for her grandson's custody arrangement. But she had always hesitated to move because of her dad and his strong ties with the community and, of course, Mike.

Jackson heard about Lavonne's dilemma and offered a novel solution: Why not have Waldo move into the spare room at Mike's house? They could both benefit by having more time together and from having the caregivers full time. After all, Waldo had difficulty with congestive heart failure and needed someone to remind him to take his medications on time and it had been a long time since he made his own dinner. Everyone, especially Mike and Waldo, agreed that this would be a good arrangement. Lavonne and Waldo gave a regular monthly amount to help pay for the caregivers, and Jackson was glad that his dad would have more company.

Lavonne and her grandson moved away and Waldo moved in with Mike. For many months, it seemed to be an ideal setup. Mike and Waldo kept each other company and the caregivers were easily able to manage the care of both. Some weekends, Lavonne would come and take Waldo for an overnight visit to her new home so that Waldo could spend time with her and his great-grandson. The daytime caregiver, Melissa, would organize an outing on the weekdays with Mike and Waldo to go to the senior center or a cafe for lunch. They would ride on the local assistive transit bus, and the "guys," as Melissa called them fondly, would strike up conversations with other older riders, talking about the changes to the town that they grew up in.

As time went on, however, Mike's dementia, now diagnosed as Alzheimer's, progressed. His episodes of confusion worsened and he began to have unusual thoughts about Waldo. He became convinced that his friend was taking money from him and would tell Melissa over and over again that she needed to check in Waldo's room for his cash. Melissa tried to assure Mike that Mike didn't keep a lot of cash in the house and that Waldo wouldn't do that to his friend. However, Melissa understood after the first few times of trying this that it would only upset Mike further, so she would just try to distract him with another activity or separate the two men in different rooms. Waldo in turn was very hurt and upset that his dear old pal would say something like this about him. A little hard of hearing, he would talk loudly to Melissa about "what in the world is wrong with Mike?" which Mike would overhear, and he would start responding angrily back. Melissa noticed that when Waldo was away from the house with his daughter, Mike was calmer and easier to manage. Finally, one day Melissa found Mike in Waldo's room standing near his friend with his fist raised, shaking with anger.

Lavonne and Jackson sadly agreed that the arrangement that had been so perfect had become a danger for both the men. Though Waldo wanted to move back with his daughter, Lavonne remained convinced that Waldo would not do well to move so far away from his hometown. Her own life situation had grown more complicated with increasing need for her attention for her grandson, who was struggling in his new setting. She wondered how she would manage to take care of both her father and her grandson on a daily basis and continue to meet the demands of her new job.

Reluctantly, Waldo agreed to go with Lavonne to find an assisted living home. The first few that they looked at gave them both a sad feeling and they felt uncertain about what to do. Then a friend told them about a good place that his mother had lived in. It was a smaller, less fancy facility, but clean and bright. It was run by a family who also owned a restaurant nearby. The owner greeted them at the door and asked a CNA to take them for a little tour. When they were looking at a possible room, the owner popped back in and asked Waldo if he would like it painted or spruced up in any way. Waldo agreed that a fresh coat of paint would make it seem brighter and they picked out a color. While the cost of the room and one month's rent deposit was more than what Waldo had been contributing toward the cost of the caregivers at Mike's, it was manageable. He was able to bring in some of his own furnishings that he had taken to Mike's house. After moving in, Waldo was soon getting to know his neighbors in the assisted living facility, enjoying the resident Labrador, and going on every outing that was offered. The nurse at the facility noticed that Waldo's blood pressure was a little high and monitored it for his doctor. Lavonne came to visit on the weekends and was pleased to see that her dad was settling in and that the care was good.

BREAKING DOWN THE COST OF HOME CARE: THE COLD HARD FACTS

As the journey unfolds for providing care for an elder, assess costs of care early in the process. For many families there comes a point at which paying for the cost of private caregivers exceeds the income and assets available. This may necessitate selling an elder's home to pay for assisted living. There are other options that you can discuss with a financial planner like home equity lines of credit or reverse mortgages. Knowing the average cost of care will help in making these difficult decisions.

According to Genworth, the average cost for private duty care from an agency in 2015 was $20 an hour. Some agencies will charge more and some will charge less, depending on the hours of care needed, region of the country, availability of staff, and whether you live in a metropolitan or rural area. If you are using an online company, costs vary there as well. With Honor.com, whose caregivers are employees of the business, consumers in the San Francisco area are charged about $30 an hour and the care provider makes between $15 and $17 an hour.[1] On Care.com, where the consumer hires directly from the website, care providers are charging between $10 and $30 an hour.

At the beginning, your elder may only need a few hours a day—let's say three to four hours for help with taking a shower, cooking, and some light housekeeping. At seven days a week averaging $20 an hour, this totals about $1,680 a month, which is over a third of the way toward the average monthly cost of an assisted living facility, which is estimated to be $3,600 a month.[2] That cost typically does not include any additional care and is considered a "base rate."

Many of you may be thinking that this is well over what you could afford anyway. As mentioned previously, there are programs that you may qualify for to assist with payment for some caregiving hours, or you may decide to hire a family member or someone else at a rate that is under the hourly cost of an agency. Just keep in mind the risks that come with hiring privately. We discuss strategies for paying for care in more detail in chapter 9.

Jack's Story

Jack is an eighty-seven-year-old man who has been relatively healthy his entire life, but diabetes and a gradual decline in his strength have taken a bit of a toll. He is widowed and lives independently in a condominium in a mid-sized city. He takes pride in his ability to manage his life, communicating with his daughter and son who live in a different state via e-mail. His daughter talks him into getting an emergency response system pendant in case he falls. He hates wearing it mainly because it labels him as being "old."

One day he falls. Jack is not wearing his emergency response pendant and lies on the floor for several hours before someone in the hall hears him crying out. The ambulance is called and he goes to the emergency room and learns he has a broken hip. Jack has hip surgery and is sent to rehab for a few weeks. When he comes home he needs help with a few activities and he hires a caregiver through a local company. At first he just needs help with some cleaning and cooking, which amounts to about two hours a day. The astute caregiver notices a sore on Jack's heel that appears to have been there for some time.

Jack goes to see his doctor, who tells Jack that this type of sore develops when someone lies in bed for an extended period of time and Jack probably didn't notice it due to his diabetes and accompanying neuropathy, which makes it difficult for him to feel pain or discomfort in his legs and feet. Jack's doctor places a boot on Jack's foot to suspend his heel and recommends not putting pressure on the heel until it is completely healed.

Now Jack needs much more help than he was getting. He has difficulty walking and also requires a nurse to come in on a regular basis to check his wound. Jack's physician puts in orders for a nurse to come to Jack's home to do wound care. Meanwhile, the private duty help he needs balloons to six hours a day seven days a week and includes help with bathing, transferring from his bed in the morning, getting dressed, and cooking more meals.

Jack decides to talk with his children about the possibility of moving to assisted living. The cost of private duty is now up to $3,500 a month and the cost is straining Jack's budget.

A change in circumstances can happen very quickly for an elder, or for anyone for that matter. You may also have had the experience of breaking a limb or getting very sick with the flu or pneumonia. Suddenly all of the activities, chores, and responsibilities that you cruised through in a day become not only more difficult, but sometimes impossible. Now imagine that you are an eighty-seven-year-old. It is not unusual for a situation to progress from several hours a day to overnight care in addition to two people needed during the day to transfer someone out of bed, onto the toilet, into the shower, or into a vehicle. That level of care would easily surpass even the cost of nursing home care, which Genworth reports to average $220 a day for a semi-private room and $250 a day for a private room. Remember, Medicare does not pay for long-term care, only short-term rehabilitation.

COMPLEXITY OF CARE

According to Genworth, the national median rate for nursing home care in a semi-private room is $220 a day. This equals about $6,600 a month. Changes with an elder can occur slowly or with a sudden cascade of events that plunge everyone into crisis mode. Sometimes it is the slow, inexorable march of dementia that erodes a person's independence and decision-making capacity.

Other times a medical event like a broken hip can snap into focus all of the other underlying medical issues that were being managed and didn't seem all that serious. Simple day-to-day tasks become momentous. Tasks like managing incontinence or a catheter, oxygen in the home, wound care, mobility problems, assistance with medication, and coping with sight impairment drive the decision making of who will do what and at what cost.

Add to the challenge of these problems the state law requirements for what an agency can and can't do. If your state restricts what an employee can do for a client (for example, they can't administer medications or manage continence care), you will have to look at other options to provide the care your elder requires in order to stay at home. Home health can fill in temporarily with services like nursing, physical therapy, and aide service for personal care tasks, but it is time limited and aides cannot provide duties like cleaning or cooking. Typically, staff from home health only come to the home three times a week on average. Here is a list of some of the more difficult tasks for a home care agency or home health to manage:

- Expensive transportation: If an elder requires wheelchair transport, this can be expensive. If you live in a rural area or smaller town, this service may not even be available.
- Two person assistance without equipment: It can be expensive and difficult to staff a situation in which two people are needed to transfer someone from bed to wheelchair, or to the bathroom, or from sitting to standing. Some agencies will insist on a transfer device due to staffing or safety issues.
- Continuous care needs that exceed the capacity of an agency or home health to be able meet. For example, daily wound treatment, catheter care, or daily insulin injections, to name a few.

- Dementia: Cognitive impairment due to dementia can be very difficult to manage in a home environment. Forgetfulness, wandering,
confusion, and waking during the night are just some of the symptoms that can be an ongoing problem, but can often be managed in
the familiar surroundings of home. Other more difficult symptoms
include aggression and sexually inappropriate behavior that can be
more difficult to manage in the home environment.

MANAGEMENT BECOMES UNMANAGEABLE

Even when there is a care agency involved, the evolving nature of aging
and health demands that you know how care is being delivered in the
home. A good care agency monitors their staff and resolves daily problems that arise. In your role as the family manager of caregiving in the
home, you may adopt varying levels of involvement. This depends largely on your relationship with the agency and their administrative staff and
the caregivers that you interact with in the home. Certainly there are some
who will trust that the agency will do what it is being paid to do. They
will assume that the care gets done properly and focus primarily on their
elder family member's health and well-being. They will stay connected
with weekly phone calls to their parent, note upcoming doctor's visits,
and have planned visits. Others will find that they want more information
on a regular if not daily basis about the care and how their family member
is responding to that care.

Not all agencies are created equal and your experience may be less
than ideal. We have heard families be told at the last minute that the night
caregiver called in sick and "you will have to cover it yourself." Another
person we know had set up cameras in the home and watched with rage as
the caregiver sat sleeping in the daytime and her mother with dementia
sat beside her with a look of total bewilderment at the stranger in her
house. Some care agencies send a different caregiver for every day, perhaps because of dealing with the very real problem of staff retention.
Whatever the reason, it makes consistent care impossible and can be very
stressful for the elder, especially if they have dementia or other cognitive
difficulties. Some agencies may have a poor system for communicating
with staff. After being as patient as you can be after a medication error

occurs, and the next day the same thing happens with a different caregiver, you may be ready to give up.

When you hire privately, you have a job as an employer with all of the responsibilities of that role. You do the hiring, firing, payroll, insurance, and oversee your employee. It is a constant, ongoing job. One of the trickiest and most stressful issues for a family caregiving manager with privately hired caregivers is when a caregiver calls in sick for a shift. Some privately hired caregivers have an informal network of others who do the same. They assist each other to cover when needed. But those are more people that you have the responsibility to assess with interviews and background checks. You may make an arrangement with a care agency to call on them when you have a hole in your schedule. This is great when it works. Remember, they have call ins too and are going to cover their schedule first over a family that is perhaps not a regular customer. Depending on your situation, you may or may not have an adequate backup plan.

If your or your parents' care grows more complicated, it may require additional caregivers. Changes in mobility usually force the decision to have one more person available for bathing and dressing. Whether you have an agency or hire privately, having more people in the home coming and going can create more need for your attention to detail.

In addition to the pressure that you may feel anticipating an early morning call about someone needing to stay home to tend to their own sick child, you will have more unexpected events. Caregivers quit for a variety of reasons, just as people do in any other field. They may graduate from college and be offered a position in their chosen field. They may get pregnant and decide that the physical requirements of the job are not good for their condition. They may move to another state with their fiancé. They may quit so that they can take care of one of their own family members full time. They may opt to go to another job that offers more hours that you have not been able to provide. Then you are back to the drawing board, scrambling in the search to find the right caregiver to help in your home or at your elder's. After you go through this routine a time or two, you may decide that it is too much in addition to all of your other responsibilities.

For a family care manager, there are parallels to the well-known plight of the family caregiver. You are not providing the hands-on 24/7 care, but you are never off duty. The management role that you have taken on is a second, usually unpaid job with unpredictable hours. These duties can intrude on other responsibilities in your life, including work hours and income. Your children's needs may be put on the back burner at times when a crisis or an urgent situation develops with your parent. Stress can become chronic and have adverse effects on your own health. It may simply become an untenable situation.

WHEN HOME ISN'T FLEXIBLE ENOUGH ANYMORE

When people are living at home and begin to realize that their needs are changing, many are able to assess their home and start making modifications. Maybe your son-in-law comes over one weekend and puts up the grab bars in the bathroom and installs a toilet seat riser for you. Other DIYs include building ramps to the front door, creating wheelchair access, or changing out door knobs for easier to use door handles. When you can afford it, you can put in stair lifts, purchase a hospital bed, or remodel a bathroom on the main floor with a roll-in shower.

What is most common is that these projects are done in dribs and drabs over time. The result may work for some phases of decline in health and mobility and not others. Some elders may not appreciate the changes to their beloved home.

Finally, especially for someone who lives in an old home, it can be like caring for an additional elder. You can add modifications for the elder person who lives there, but what about the ancient plumbing that is now dripping through the living room ceiling? If you notice the lights flickering regularly, does it mean that you are able to afford to dig out the wiring to update and repair it? Some elders have not done much to downsize. For some who have the issue of hoarding, the home becomes high risk for safety concerns such as increasing falls, being hit on the head or shoulders by falling debris, and the whole home can be a fire hazard. We know one elder hoarder whose home was declared a disaster area after a leaking pipe was undetected due to massive clutter in her basement. The leak flooded that level and the first floor (only passable by narrow paths between mountains of stuff), making it unlivable.

The old home place might just not be what it used to be. It might not be possible for you to find the finances, not to mention the time, to be a part-time contractor to make it feasible as an ongoing home environment.

ASSISTED LIVING: PANACEA OR PREDICAMENT?

When families and elders think of assisted living, all kinds of ideas and expectations come to mind. Some of these are accurate, some are wishful thinking, and some are completely erroneous. Countless times we have heard elders speak about assisted living as if it is a nursing home—a doomed place that conjures images of very sick and disabled people receiving constant nursing care. Other images reflect the marketing brochures that show vibrant, gray-haired people sitting on a patio sipping tea or playing croquet on a manicured lawn. Assisted living can be a viable option for many families, but being educated about what is available in your state and what the costs are can help you make an informed decision about whether it makes sense to give up caregivers for assisted living.

It isn't often that people really take stock of what an assisted living community can and can't do. Just like our previous section on what tasks a private duty caregiver can perform depending on the state they work in, assisted living rules and regulations vary according to state. What this means is that each state will dictate what kind of care they can provide and when they can legally request that a resident move to a higher level of care, which is typically a nursing home. The term assisted living is somewhat generic in that many states have varying degrees of residential care with different requirements for each level. As an elder or family member considering assisted living, it will be helpful to know what is available in your state so you can be assured that the care provided is actually what is needed. Depending on what your options are, you may have to augment care with private duty anyway.

New York, for example, has these designations for residential care: (please refer to the National Center for Assisted Living 2016 state regulatory review for more specific information): [3]

- Adult care facility: Family-type home for adults that provides temporary or long-term residential care for adults who are by reason of physical or other limitations unable to live independently and do not require continual medical or nursing care.
- Adult home: A type of adult care facility that provides long-term residential care, room, board, housekeeping, personal care, and supervision to five or more adults.

- Enriched housing program: A type of adult care facility that provides long-term residential care to five or more adults (generally sixty-five years of age or older) in community-integrated settings resembling independent housing units and provides or arranges for room, board, housekeeping, personal care, and supervision. Units in these homes have a kitchenette.
- Assisted living and an assisted living residence: A type of adult care facility that is licensed as an adult home or enriched housing program and provides the highest level of care. These operators may also be certified as special needs assisted living to provide dementia care or as enhanced assisted living to support aging in place. These homes provide or arrange for housing, on-site monitoring, and personal care and/or home care services, either directly or indirectly, in a home-like setting for five or more adults unrelated to the assisted living provider.
- Enhanced assisted living: For residents who are unable to walk with assistance or require another person to walk. They are dependent on medical equipment and may have chronic unmanaged urinary or bowel incontinence.
- Special needs assisted living (called memory care in some states) for people with special needs.
- Assisted living program: Serves private pay and Medicaid-eligible individuals who are medically eligible for nursing home placement, but who are not in need of the highly structured medical environment of a nursing facility and whose needs could be met in a less restrictive and lower-cost residential setting.

Now compare New York with the State of New Mexico. New Mexico has one designation: assisted living.

Unfortunately, the consumer cannot always choose the level of care they want to be in and there are rules that may exclude some people from certain types of facilities. For example, some states require that residents be able to vacate the building on their own, which would mean that they can't be substantially bed bound. According to a 2010 report from the Center for Disease Control, 59 percent of residential care facilities did not admit a person who requires two people to transfer them or who need specialized transfer equipment, such as a Hoyer lift, to get them in and out of bed.[4]

In many cases, the presented cost of assisted living is a base rate and care costs are added on. These add-on costs typically correspond to "levels of care." The level of care will determine the additional add-on cost per month. Level of assistance is assessed in these general domains:

- Bathing: Can a person bathe independently or do they need assistance and how often?
- Dressing: How much assistance does a person need to get dressed and undressed?
- Grooming: Shaving, brushing teeth and hair.
- Mobility: Can the resident walk? Do they need assistance with getting out of bed or from sitting to standing?
- Continence: Can the person manage their own continence supplies or do they need reminders or someone to actually change them?
- Caregivers: Sometimes two care providers are needed for agitated or combative residents when they are bathing.
- Eating: Some people have swallowing problems and need a care provider to sit with them to monitor their eating.
- Medications: Many assisted living communities group medications into the number of medications that have to be administered and assign a level based on that number. Does the person need injections?
- Laundry: Some assisted living communities include laundry in their base rate, but some charge.
- Dementia: People with dementia require more care. They may wander or become agitated or inappropriate and therefore there will be an add-on cost.

When investigating assisted living facilities, make sure the add-on costs are thoroughly explained. If your elder is considering assisted living, a nurse should come to wherever the elder is and do an assessment and base costs on the results of that assessment. Once in assisted living, expect costs to go up each year, and expect that the level of care may increase as well.

The biggest problem with assisted living? It isn't home. Although the advantages look good on paper, many people would rather stay at home paying for and managing the care that they need, rather than move to assisted living or other congregate housing. However, there are many examples of successful moves from home care to assisted living.

Marilyn and Larry

Marilyn and Larry are a couple in their eighties who live alone in their own home. Both Marilyn and Larry have memory problems and Larry also has depression that contributes to him spending most of the day in bed. Marilyn and Larry's children live out of town and are too busy with their own lives to provide any support. The one thing that Marilyn and Larry's children do is contact a personal care agency who sends a care provider over three days a week to do some cooking and laundry.

Marilyn feels increasingly overwhelmed at the obligations she has at the house, and Larry defers to her for all decision making. Larry is no longer able to drive, so all of the driving is left to Marilyn, and she has become increasingly uncomfortable with her driving skills. The home is cluttered and needs a great deal of maintenance. Larry has a hospital bed in the living room surrounded by clutter and debris. Marilyn mentions to the care provider that she would like to consider an assisted living community. The care provider agrees to take Marilyn to visit a few and Marilyn decides on one. She arranges to sell their modest home and they move.

Marilyn and Larry must now share a small studio room, which is quite an adjustment from their large house, but a studio is all they can afford. The staff at the assisted living community are welcoming and supportive. Although their room is small, there are common areas such as a library and lobby with large sofa chairs and there is a large dining room. The activities director is instrumental in engaging Marilyn in activities, and although Larry doesn't really participate, he feels comforted by the activity around him. Marilyn begins to venture out and make friends. Driving is no longer an issue because transportation is provided by the assisted living community.

After a few months, Larry's health deteriorates and he goes to a nursing home, where he eventually dies. Marilyn is able to move to a larger room and continues to engage with other residents and activities. A physician visits the community on a regular basis and sees to Marilyn's medical needs.

Marilyn eventually runs out of funds to pay for assisted living, but the resident advocate helps her apply for state assistance and she happily is able to stay.

MEMORY CARE: SHOP WISELY

In our work with elders, we have been excited to see changes in the care of people with dementia over the last two decades. While there is much research required to find a way to prevent these debilitating conditions, there is also much study of what constitutes good care for people with dementia. There is more thought going into what types of physical and social environments truly create a healthy living setting for someone with these progressive conditions.

Unfortunately, there are many residential facilities that tout their specialty memory care units that have only a superficial gloss and not much else.[5] Sadly, we have seen some of these units be nothing more than a locked unit that only serves to segregate people with any signs of dementia from the general resident group.

It is important to keep in mind a few realities of dementia as you shop wisely for the right memory care facility for a family member suffering from one of these disorders:

- A person with dementia is very sensitive to changes in their environment and at certain stages, seek familiarity for reassurance. The transition to a new living environment must be handled very carefully.
- A specialty memory care unit cannot stop the progression of the disease. However, a good memory care unit can support your goal for your loved one to live in an appropriately stimulating environment and maintain their peace of mind and dignity.

As many as 70 percent of people with dementia live at home, usually with mild to moderate forms of the disease.[6] However, there are growing numbers of people with dementia residing in senior care homes of all varieties. According to the Alzheimer's Association, there are currently 64 percent of nursing home residents in this country who have dementia and 42 percent of residents of assisted living homes have it.[7]

Memory care units are an expanding sector of the economy.[8] The memory care industry reports an increasing uptick in demand, according to the National Investment Center for Seniors Housing and Care, or NIC, a not-for-profit organization based in Annapolis, Maryland. Their data indicate that as of 2016, "there are about 12,200 units under construction."[9] These new facilities, about two thirds of which are add-ons to an existing senior housing, tout "evidence-based design" and beautiful decor. This construction boom raises numerous questions, including: Will these units be affordable? Will they really make a difference in the quality of care for the resident or is it simply more appealing to the younger relatives arranging the care? Who is staffing these units? What kind of training do they have? And with the fierce competition for the best caregivers, how will these units attract them?

The cost of entering a specialty memory care unit will vary in different states. In 2015, the extra fees attached to these units over the average cost of assisted living or a nursing home were approximately an additional $1,200 month.[10]

As you shop for one, note what services and themes they have on offer and compare them with other memory care units. For example:

- What is the staff to resident ratio? What efforts are made to keep the same staff with one resident? More staff and consistent care is essential for memory care.
- Look for a safe but nonthreatening design (no bars or loud buzzers when doors open and close).
- Attention to nutrition and wellness.
- Memory-specific therapeutic and social programs on the calendar.
- Look at ways that the unit prevents the elder with dementia from becoming isolated.
- Seek a program that has a stated goal to use medications in the least restrictive way possible.

Perhaps the most important factor in any memory care scenario is the human element. Of course, you want to have people in these "hands-on" roles be kind and motivated to provide good, person-centered care. You want their training and understanding of dementia to be up to date and inclusive. Individual states determine the types of training for dementia care and the number of hours required for assisted living and nursing home memory care units. For instance, for assisted living staff, many states have a specific dementia training curriculum, some have competency examinations, and most have specific hourly training requirements for employees on these units both before and usually after they are on the job.[11] There are only some states that do not require special dementia training for assisted living staff (Alaska, Hawaii, Maryland, Michigan, North Dakota, Ohio, and Puerto Rico). Do ask at each facility how they conduct training and if and how staff get continuing education.

AN INTERVIEW WITH A DAUGHTER

What was your father's life like when he was living at home with caregivers?

Dad had live-in care for almost four years. He had two male caregivers that split the week living with him. Several years prior we had done many of the typical safety things: we added bars to the bathroom (in the shower and by the toilet), purchased a shower chair for him to sit in, added "no skid" materials to the several stairs he had to take to get out to the garage (and added a railing for these stairs). We had also added deadbolts on all doors (dad had vascular dementia—and didn't wander like many with Alzheimer's are known to do—but he did once go out into the garage and got in the car while his care person was in the shower. He didn't have the keys, but it still concerned us).

But they were beginning to struggle caring for him alone. He was struggling with increasing incontinence and other issues that made it more challenging for a live-in care person alone. Another thing that concerned me was his increasing isolation—as his disease progressed, fewer people visited him and of course he went out less (he did go to church every Sunday up until his move—his care person would take him). I was beginning to think that a facility would provide more stimulation for him.

How did it become clear that living at home with caregivers was no longer working? Was there a "straw that broke the camel's back" event or just a realization that it was no longer working?

As is common, my father had an event that forced a decision. He broke his hip. He didn't need surgery—but did need to go into a rehab facility for two months, with one month in a wheelchair (putting no pressure on his hip) and then a month of physical therapy. He did remarkably well in rehab and walked out of the facility—but we used this event as an opportunity to transition him to a memory care facility. While it was an "event"—we knew that he was a fall risk, and our family home wasn't set up for a wheelchair (it would have required substantial changes to the house) and it wasn't even easier for a walker. We thought going from rehab to the assisted living might be easier for him than going back to his home for a short period of time and then relocating him. It was still a difficult transition for him—on the drive to the memory care facility (directly from the rehab facility) when I didn't turn at one intersection (toward his home) he asked me why I didn't turn. It was heartbreaking. I hadn't thought he would remember the turn.

How did you find the facility that you chose?

I toured seven facilities. Honestly, it was a hard decision because personally I didn't like any of them—I wanted my father to be cared for at home, but I had to accept that it was no longer practical.

The facility we chose was all on one floor and was small. Because it was small it had fewer added features, but I liked that it was small and in a more rural setting. The window in many of the rooms looked over a green space, and there was a sweet (fenced/secured) garden in the rear of the facility as well. At the time I was still spending quite a bit of time in my home in another state, and so it was important for the facility to be close to my dad's two younger brothers. The facility I chose was between ten and fifteen minutes from their homes—and they visited him frequently (for the first two years, one of them visited each day—mostly alternating days). He was in the facility for three and a half years, and I moved back for most of the last two years.

Were you happy with the care that your dad had there, or were there ongoing issues that concerned you?

There were ongoing issues. I was a very involved advocate. It was an "assisted living" memory care facility—so not a skilled nursing facility. They do support "aging in place," which I liked, although later I learned that because they weren't a skilled nursing facility that they weren't as qualified to handle certain situations.

Over the course of three and a half years I called the facility's corporate headquarters three times—mostly related to staffing concerns (insufficient staff on duty).

What is your list of positives and negatives?

Something I had to get used to was the turnover in staff. I would get used to a care provider or a group of them, and then they would leave—I felt like I was constantly sharing the same information about my dad to staff on a regular basis. We also had three different facility directors over a three-and-a-half-year period—and each were different with respect to what they felt was important and how they staffed the facility. Each change brings adjustments. When my father was admitted, I filled out numerous forms that I took quite seriously—personal details about my dad that would facilitate his care. Generally I felt like everyone was winging it and that no one really took the time to look it over (other than details related to meds and allergies).

I tend to be an "it takes a village" person—and that a facility is only as good as the advocates/family members are—that is, advocates strengthen the facilities and keep them honest and on task. It was surprising to me how hands-off many family members were—it was as if once their family member was admitted, they didn't feel that they needed to continue caring for their family member, that everything was taken care of. Many took a hands-off approach—they would visit, but they weren't involved. When you tour a place, I would advise to go at different times, and perhaps times when family might be visiting—do they seem like they are visiting a casual acquaintance or just watching—or do they seem involved in what is going on? The more family that are dedicated to staying involved the better the facility will be.

Communication between staff was generally not good. Things that would be extremely important to me (so something critical to my dad's care or quality of life) were most often insufficiently communicated. I often felt like staff had a minimal checklist in their heads for what they needed to do for each individual, and they often went through that checklist without thoroughly assessing the resident. They felt like they had done their "job" if they completed the minimal checklist—and they often didn't look outside of that list for other things that might need to be done.

What worked for your dad and what didn't?

I hired someone to visit with dad from 11 a.m. until 2 p.m. each day. I was fortunate and found young people (ranging in age from fifteen to twenty-six) over the three-and-a-half-year period who did things with him that the staff didn't have time to do or didn't do frequently enough for me. This included taking him outside whenever the weather was nice, doing arts and crafts with him, reading books to him, working on his reading and the alphabet and cognitive exercises, engaging him (and later assisting him) during lunch and in essence being an extra set of eyes for me. I was fortunate to have found delightful and dedicated individuals—one young woman was with my father for three years (Monday through Friday for three hours a day) and another young woman was with him for one and a half years (Saturday through Sunday for three hours a day). They became his close friends and provided continuity for him since the staff frequently changed.

I worked hard to learn what "extra" care was available—and covered by insurance for him. This was not immediately known to me—but I discovered that his memory care assisted living facility was connected to excellent "home health" staff—physical therapists, occupational therapists, and speech (swallow) therapists. I took advantage of these services as often as I could—they provided engagement, therapy, and another set of eyes on my dad. It made me wish there was a comprehensive checklist for caregivers of those dealing with dementia. I've often thought of writing a guidebook myself, from the perspective of a family member/advocate/guardian.

I got to know all the administrative staff well. Every time there was someone new, I introduced myself. I visited six days a week for almost two years. I also volunteered at the facility and for the last year coordinated a concert for the residents. I have no doubt that a resident with a more involved family member will receive better care. I visited at different times every day. But although I'm sure that I was considered a demanding family member by the care providers/staff—they also knew that I was committed and pulled my own weight by chipping in when needed and by running the concert series that benefited all residents.

What is your advice to someone who is looking for memory care after they have decided living at home is not an option?

Be sure to look beyond how nice the lobby is, or how nice the person giving you the tour is—they are salespeople and will only provide you with positive spin. After your family member moves in, they have little to no involvement with your family member—so they are essentially the least important people with respect to your parent's actual care.

The people that matter most are the staff—the care providers—who also are the lowest paid employees at the facility. These are the people that got my dad up in the morning, that showered him, that helped him with his meals and dressed him. When you visit a facility, pay attention to these people and what they are doing: Are they looking at residents in the eye? Are they touching them? Are they smiling or do they seem stressed and unhappy? Are they busy or lingering in the hallway or smoking outside as you walk in? Are they being kind, and talking to the residents in a calm or sweet voice—and not sounding frustrated or angry?

How many care providers are there per resident? What is their level of training? You can ask these questions to the person giving you a tour, but I'd also ask to speak with the head of the nursing staff and the director and see how well their answers correlate to one another. Also, try to visit several times and at different times—what is the atmosphere during meal time, or early in the morning or mid-afternoon?

Has the activity director been trained in activities for those with dementia? How much training did they receive? How long has the activities director been there? When you first get there, check out the activities calendar—do they seem to actually be doing the activities listed? Quite often they make this calendar look festive and busy—but often they can't sustain that schedule—so check to see if the activities listed are realistic, appropriate, and sufficiently challenging for someone with cognitive challenges.

Talk to the physician that is responsible for residents at the facility. Make sure you like him or her. For the first year we retained my father's geriatric physician—but it became more difficult as his disease progressed to drive into town for appointments, so the in-house doctor became his primary physician during the period when he was in decline. Get to know this physician and the nursing staff—too often they come in, meet with your family member when you aren't there, and you receive secondhand information from the facility nurse that can be confusing or incomplete. *Always follow up* if you have a question.

Remember that what is urgent to you is not always as urgent to the staff. If you are sure that it is urgent, then push it (tests for UTIs [or urinary tract infections], for example, should be pushed—they can become serious quickly). Don't ever hesitate to follow up with anyone about anything.

Personally, I think folks with dementia are always underestimated—by staff, by physicians, by administrators, and by family. Everyone is constantly monitoring them for declining cognition—and in the process, they fail to engage what remains. In my father's facility, only the very late-stage individuals were hard to engage, and even sometimes they would respond.

FEARS AND FEELINGS ABOUT MOVING AWAY FROM HOME

There's no doubt that it is not the top choice for many people to move from home to a senior residence. People may have looked ahead when they were younger and made the decision: "Not for me!" Time catches up and suddenly you may be facing the inevitability of a move to a senior home. For many, it is a time of emotional turmoil. People have legitimate feelings of sadness, hopelessness, loss, anxiety, and even anger. Some of these feelings are also experienced by the adult children and family members. There is a grieving of loss of the life lived at the home.

Here are some of the common reactions that we hear from elders about moving to senior care:

1. "I've visited friends at these places. Everyone there has dementia."
2. "There are only old people there."
3. "I'm not a joiner. I like my time by myself. I don't want to play Bingo all day."
4. "My home is a part of me. I can't possibly leave."
5. "I would feel lonesome without my neighborhood and friends."
6. "I will only get older and sicker in one of these places."

While the online marketing of the senior housing industry will assure you that these feelings are based on myths, it is unwise not to listen and discuss these real feelings of the elder and of other family members. There is research and evidence that a large number of elders do in fact decline after a move to a nursing home. [12]

The fear of the unknown is a large part of people's negative attitudes about moving from a beloved home and senior living. Taking the elder along for assessing the options for their new living environment is an absolute must unless it is completely impossible, such as for medical reasons. A very good strategy for a successful outcome is to try a respite stay at a chosen facility. Many senior residences offer this opportunity. A senior can stay at a facility for a defined time, usually a number of weeks. Some families do this when a family caregiver is going on a vacation or other travel or simply needs a break from caregiving duties.

Magrit's Story

Magrit grew up as a teenager in Nazi Germany in a small village. It was a difficult and traumatic time and the postwar years were equally horrendous with food shortages, the destruction that ravaged the country, and mourning the loss of many of her family killed in the war itself. Magrit remembers feeling lost and trapped at the same time. It was no wonder that when given the opportunity, Magrit moved away from her home country as a young adult, hiding her German heritage from neighbors as she relocated to other countries. When she made her way to a new continent, finding work as a waitress in a small town in Wyoming, she insinuated that she was originally from Austria to avoid anti-German sentiment common in the United States after the war. She slowly made a life for herself there. She met and married a wonderful man, became a U.S. citizen, had several children, and they moved many places in the states and in South America with her husband's career as a geologist. Many decades later, they settled in Montana, planning a life of active retirement. Unfortunately, early in this phase of their life Magrit's husband suffered from a heart condition and died relatively young. Magrit became depressed after his death and struggled to overcome that difficult condition. In time, she regained her strength and began to explore what this unexpected widowhood would mean for her. She became an advocate for others who suffered with depression. She was determined that after surviving more pain in her life she would make this part of her life a success. She began to celebrate her age with brightly colored clothes and enjoyed wearing big earrings and a bigger smile.

Magrit was becoming active in the senior center in her town and going on jaunts with others to museums and local events. She became a volunteer at the local library. She began to notice a feeling of not feeling quite herself and started to have overpowering vertigo. She was assessed at a balance clinic and her doctors concluded that she had a rare balance condition that would progress and worsen. They advised her to consider moving into an assisted living facility. The thought of this horrified Magrit. After all, she had always been active, hiking and exploring the beautiful outdoors with her husband and children in the different mountainous regions where they had lived. The suggestion of it gave her that trapped feeling that she knew only too well from her early life.

Magrit's daughter who lived nearby supported her decision to stay at home. She did errands for Magrit such as grocery and supply shopping and would spend the weekends at her mother's to care for her. At first, Magrit proudly maintained as much activity as she could. Because she couldn't drive anymore, she learned to take the local support transit. She continued to volunteer at the library for very short hours and the library accommodated her needs by making her job to sit at the main reference desk to field phone calls and assist patrons there. When she struggled to dress and bathe independently, she hired a local caregiver three mornings a week to help her. In her view, these were small sacrifices to make to ensure that she could maintain her freedom.

Over the following year, however, the vertigo worsened. She suffered from syncope or fainting due to a sudden drop in her blood pressure. She would regain consciousness soon after, finding herself on the floor. As these episodes increased and the doctors were unable to control the changes in her blood pressure, her daughter became increasingly alarmed. She and Magrit discussed the idea of the two of them living together to increase Magrit's safety. Neither lived in a place big enough for Magrit, her daughter, and her daughter's ten-year-old son. They looked at moving from each of their homes to a third bigger place. The financial questions for this option were complicated for Magrit's daughter. While they were trying to figure out how to make this work, Magrit had a fall at her home when she was by herself that resulted in a broken shoulder. She ended up in the hospital. She decided that she did not want to infringe on her daughter's freedom. When the hospital discharge care manager came to talk to her, they talked about an assisted living facility. They found one that agreed to allow her to live there on the condition that she always use a walker like a Rollator with a handy seat, so that she could sit quickly if vertigo or fainting appeared imminent.

While the move was uneventful, Magrit was despondent about her new living quarters. Though she took as many personal furnishings as she could fit into her studio apartment at the assisted living home, it still felt cold and institutional to her. She hated the regimented schedule of activities. But most of all, she felt that she did not belong there. Though in her early seventies, she felt much younger in spirit than the other residents. She felt the burden of her medical condition more acutely. There were even people older than herself there who had more mobility. She had a fall in her room, but hid this from the staff and her daughter, fearing that if they found out they would insist that she move to a nursing home.

Magrit's depression returned. She became hopeless, lethargic, and withdrawn. She stayed awake nights missing her old home, thinking of it as the last connection she had had with her deceased husband. Her appetite became inconsistent and she became more negative and irritable, complaining about the food at the assisted living home as being not fit for consumption. In fact, Magrit began to complain about everything about the place, from the staff being nincompoops to the other residents as being a bunch of gossipy old people. Magrit's daughter realized that this was not simply a matter of her mother having a difficult transition to her new home. She recognized how similar this was to her mother's previous bout with depression and insisted that Magrit go back to see her therapist. Magrit began to see her therapist on a regular basis and went to a geriatric psychiatrist to have her antidepressants assessed and adjusted.

It was many months before Magrit's mood stabilized and her depression was under control. Though her depression was controlled, her view of living in the residential care remained negative. She strove to complain less because she wasn't fond of complainers. In sessions with her therapist, she considered ways to accept her fate. She was able to recognize that her current life felt at times so much like how she had survived as a child during the Nazi regime. However, now it was her own body and health that betrayed her and took her liberty from her. She tried to work through her anger and remorse. It continued to be difficult for her to move on from feeling trapped.

TAKEAWAY POINTS FOR THIS CHAPTER

- Assess current and future costs of care early in the game. Know when care costs exceed the ability of you or your elder to financially sustain care in the home.
- Know what tasks caregivers can and can't do in your state so you can fill in the gaps with other resources.
- If you are managing caregivers in the home, assess the time it takes and your own level of stress as the situation becomes more complex.
- Evaluate residential care options along with costs in your state so you can be prepared to make decisions quickly if needed. Recognize that there is the possibility that a residential care community may not accept someone due to state restrictions.
- When considering memory care, evaluate staff to resident ratio, nutrition and wellness programs, social activities, and environmental design. Be sensitive to the enormous psychological and emotional impact a move to an assisted living or memory care facility can have on an elder.

9

CREATIVE SOLUTIONS

More Than One Way Home

INTRODUCTION

The current state and future of caregiving is by necessity undergoing tremendous change. In this chapter, we are going to look at creative solutions that address how we can improve aging in community and examine some new models and ideas. We will explore how some families are thinking outside the box to manage the costs of home care. Some ideas come from the past and some from a wide array of people, professions, and industries that can make the difference for someone aging at home with care.

MODELS OF CARE THAT WORK

We'll review some current models of care that include staying in one's own home with coordinated care or moving to a small home-like residential setting with a small group of other elders with all-inclusive care. A consideration with any of these models is the challenge of increasing care needs as someone ages in place. Some of these community models are not equipped to handle complex medical problems that may necessitate someone having to move to assisted living, rehab, or a nursing home.

The Veteran's Administration Medical Foster Home Program

The Veteran's Administration Medical Foster Home Program is a simple, effective solution for elders who want to avoid nursing home care. Medical foster homes are private homes in which a trained caregiver provides services to a few individuals. Some, but not all, residents are veterans. The VA inspects and approves all medical foster homes.

A medical foster home can serve as an alternative to a nursing home. It may be appropriate for veterans who require nursing home care but prefer a noninstitutional setting with fewer residents.

Medical foster homes have at least one trained caregiver on duty twenty-four hours a day, seven days a week. This caregiver can help the veteran carry out activities of daily living, such as bathing and getting dressed. The VA ensures that the caregiver is well trained to provide VA planned care. While living in a medical foster home, veterans receive home-based primary care services.

We have observed this program firsthand, and like any program, it is only as good as the people that are providing the care. The way the program works is that a person or family applies to the VA to become a site for the Medical Foster Home Program. Some families have room for just one occupant, others have room for more. They must pass inspections, have training, and the elder veteran must be a part of the VA-sponsored Home Based Primary Care Program. This piece of the program is critical to its success. The VA Home Based Primary Care Program sends nurse practitioners, nurses, social workers, and therapy staff to the home to provide medical care. The idea is to minimize travel to the closest VA medical center for treatment and in some cases to avert medical crises by intervening sooner. The elder pays between $1,500 and $3,000 a month to live in this home setting depending on the level of care they need and financial resources.

If we deconstruct the ideas of the VA Medical Foster Home Program there are components of the program that are already in place and generating discussion across the country. The two main pieces of the program that are already being replicated are living in someone else's home and medical care provided in that home.

INTERVIEW WITH A VETERAN'S ADMINISTRATION MEDICAL FOSTER HOME CAREGIVER

How did you become interested in this program?

I was trained as a physical therapy assistant and my husband was going to school and we wanted to raise a family. This way we could stay at home while earning income. We actually remodeled our basement with the program criteria in mind. The VA requires a certification process to be a part of the program. FBI background checks, CPR and first aid, and two trainings twice a year are required with the program. An application must be submitted and a health certificate from a primary care physician must be obtained saying that you are physically capable of doing the work. The home has to meet building code to be eligible for the program. We did have to add a stair lift and ladder in the window wells for safe evacuation during an emergency. Windows have to serve as escape.

How critical do you think the Home Based Primary Care program is to the success of this program?

Home-based primary care is critical to the success of the program. It would be very difficult for the program to work without the medical personnel coming to the home. If you have to take veterans to every appointment, it would be a challenge. With the Home Based Primary Care Program they don't have to get out of the house. I still have to take veterans for specialty appointments or emergency visits, but it easier on all of us if having to drive to medical appointments is minimized. A similar program could be run without the home-based primary care but it wouldn't be as good.

You say that you have hired private caregivers to assist you with the care of your veterans. How does that work?

Hired private caregivers have to go through the same paperwork as we did. The FBI background check is no longer required, but everything else has to be completed: CPR, TB test, and training. I can hire any caregiver I want and I pay them. My experience with caregivers has been about one in three is good. The caregiver's expertise and knowledge has to be just as good as mine. I started with an online company but my experience with caregivers through the online company was not good. And the online company was horribly expensive. People didn't show for appointments or said they had a car and didn't. Now I use a local classified section and find much better caregivers that way. They make more and I pay less and the quality of person was far better. I have people calling and e-mailing me their resumes wanting the job. I have much more success with just the local online jobs posted section. Of course, I have the extra protection of the VA requirements that any caregiver must go through. The caregiver pays their own taxes. I get an exempt form that they fill out. Plus the caregivers can perform whatever tasks I can perform: administer medications, take blood pressure, perform some injections like an insulin shot, do blood sugar checks, and empty catheter and change catheter bags. It is only skilled nursing tasks like changing a catheter or drawing blood that we can't do. A nurse has to perform those tasks and that is where the Home Based Primary Care Program comes in. If the task does not require certification, myself or a caregiver can perform the task. Using a private caregiver, I pay less and they make more.

What is the biggest challenge of the program?

The biggest challenge for the veteran is being able to afford the program. For me, it is the emergency care and pop-up appointments that can be challenging to manage. But in case of emergency I also have the VA medical team I can call for advice or if they are available on short notice they can come over to evaluate one of my veterans. If the veteran has Medicare then they can receive physical therapy.

What is the best part of the program?

The best part of the program is the quality of life my veterans have. When I place my veterans in respite (a short, temporary stay) in a nursing home while I am out of town, it never goes well. They are ignored, the staff make mistakes with their medications. Every time they come back with more problems. When vets are in the VA Medical Foster Home program they do better, they live longer, and they are happier.

What do your residents do during the day?

They watch TV and read. We take them shopping or on scenic rides. If they want to go to the local senior center we take them there as well. Our hired caregiver also does activities like playing cards.

Do you think a program like this could be replicated outside the VA system?

The most difficult part of the program to replicate would be figuring out how to pay for it and provide the home-based primary care as part of the program. If those pieces could be figured out, then I think many people would be willing to host elderly or disabled people in their homes.

Residential Care Homes or Board and Care

We talked in chapter 6 about the variety of residential care licenses across the country. Some states have a diverse offering of residential care for elders and others are more restricted. For example, in the state of Washington the term is adult family home, in which a residence is licensed for up to six individuals.[1] Why consider a board and care community? Several reasons. Most board and care communities are in a residential home with many fewer residents than assisted living. This may be more appealing to your elder than a larger, more institutional setting. The second reason to consider board and care is the cost, which is typically less than assisted living. In California, the average cost of assisted living is from $1,500 to $4,500 depending on care needs. Board and care ranges from $2,500 for a shared room to $3,500 for a private room.[2] That difference in cost can free up funds to supplement care by hiring a private caregiver to take the elder on additional outings or engage in recreational activities, such as going to the senior center, shopping, or sightseeing.

Tom's Story

Tom is a seventy-year-old veteran who served in the Vietnam War. He suffered a nervous breakdown when he was in the service, but managed to finish out his tour of duty and moved into a rental home in a mid-sized city where some of his military buddies lived. Tom suffered from PTSD symptoms, which in those days was something most military personnel were just beginning to hear about but not necessarily understand, and treatment options were limited.

As time went on, Tom went from job to job and his mental health deteriorated. As his mental condition worsened, so did his physical condition. He started drinking and smoking more and generally ignoring any health concerns, even though his health care was paid for at the nearby Veteran's Medical Center. He was anxious and paranoid. Tom's home became the party house for other veterans and some people he didn't even know. His belongings began disappearing and the home became trashed. Tom's two sisters and brother had given up on trying to help him because their efforts were rebuffed.

One day Tom collapsed and a friend who was at the home called 911. Tom was taken to the emergency department at the Veteran's Medical Center where it was discovered he had chronic obstructive pulmonary disease, possible esophageal cancer, high blood pressure, malnutrition, and dehydration. An endoscopy was done with a biopsy and the results were inconclusive. It was recommended that the procedure be repeated in three months. A VA social worker recommended nursing home placement for Tom because it was unlikely he would follow through with the healthcare recommendations made by the medical team. Tom was placed in a nursing home that was contracted with the VA, and Tom was able to live there with the VA paying his expenses.

Medically, Tom began to improve with adequate food and fluids and monitoring by the nursing home staff. However, he became more and more isolated, only coming out of his room to smoke in the common smoking area. The activities director tried and tried to get him involved in activities and he always refused. Tom began to lose the weight he had put back on and became more and more depressed. He started to have the problem of urinary retention and a catheter was placed, which was a further humiliation—having to deal with a bag full of urine.

Another social worker at the nursing home, Cammie, was worried about Tom's mental health and the impact it was having on his physical health. She made a radical suggestion. Why not let Tom try living in an adult family home. The nursing home staff were adamant in their belief that Tom was incapable of functioning in such an independent environment. Cammie decided to give it a try.

Tom and Cammie visited four different adult family homes. The cost of each home was close to the VA pension that Tom received each month, but with careful budgeting he could swing it. Tom decided on a home somewhat outside the city in a more rural area. There were three other men at the home, and there was a sitting patio with a common kitchen. To Cammie's chagrin but Tom's delight, he could smoke outside. Ralph, who managed the home, was a "tinkerer" and had a couple of motorcycles in the garage that he was working on. That sealed the deal. Tom used to ride a Harley. Tom moved in.

Within two months of moving in, Tom had made friends with the resident cat and was coming out of his room and starting to come out of his shell. Cammie was shocked when Tom announced he wanted to stop smoking with a nicotine patch. Cammie arranged to get him a supply through the VA and Tom stopped smoking. The next month Tom announced that he would like to be trained to catheterize himself so he could get rid of the in-dwelling catheter. He was told he would have to self-catheterize three times a day and use sterile technique to avoid infection. Tom agreed and learned to master the technique. Tom asked Cammie to reach out to his family so he could reunite with them. Although they said they would come visit, their busy lives prevented them from making much of an effort to visit Tom. Tom asked Cammie to teach him how to ride transit and once he learned, he was able to go visit his sister that lived closest independently.

Remember Doctor House Calls?

You may be too young to remember the days when getting sick meant calling the doctor who came to the house. In a *New York Times* article by Tina Rosenberg titled "Reviving House Calls by Doctors," she writes, "Before 1950, nearly half of all doctors' visits in America were house calls. But then the country began building big hospitals and luxurious doctors' offices, and doctors acquired sophisticated equipment they couldn't put in a medical bag. Medicare and Medicaid reimbursement systems made home visits untenable. There is a slowly growing movement to bring primary care to the home, and other residential care communities."[3] A frail older person going to the doctor takes time and effort. Often a relative needs to take time off from work to get an elder to an appointment, or a caregiver takes the person. We have observed situations in which several different family members pitch in to take an elder to various doctors' appointments and confusion ensues as the communication between family members and medical providers becomes disjointed.

Moreover, if an older person lands in the hospital it costs more—an average of $1,200 per person.[4] Anything that keeps a person at home is a benefit to everyone. A physician or nurse practitioner coming to the home can observe the environment, look for fall hazards, and check on medication compliance, among other things. Elders with dementia don't get as confused when a doctor comes to their home as they do when they have to go out to see a provider. It is well worth investigating if this is an option in your area.

Another innovative program along the lines of house call doctors is Community Paramedicine.[5] The idea behind this program is that paramedics are called to an elder's home for a variety of reasons, but falls are a big one. The norm when 911 is called is to take the person to the emergency room for a complete workup, which sometimes leads to hospitalization. Hospital stays are associated with an increase in infections and delirium, not to mention the stress and confusion that accompanies a trip to the emergency room. The Community Paramedicine Program sends a trained paramedic to an elder's home to assess whether or not the person really needs to go to the hospital, and treatment is provided at the home, often avoiding a costly trip to the hospital. The program is currently operating in thirty-three different states across the country.[6]

INNOVATIVE OPTIONS FOR AGING IN PLACE

There are many exciting and creative models being developed across the country in an effort to assist elders remain independent, but with built-in support and community. Beth Baker's wonderful book *With a Little Help from Our Friends: Creating Community as We Grow Older* provides a comprehensive look at each of these models. [7] We highly recommend this book as a resource on aging in place concepts across the country. There are expensive models, but affordable ones as well. Because many of these concepts are not "advertised," knowing what they are will help you investigate their availability in your community. We will briefly summarize a few here.

The Villages

The Village to Village network began in Boston in 2002 with the idea of fostering a group of like-minded people in a geographic area who come together to figure out and develop the resources they will need to age comfortably in their own homes without moving. The villages use the strategy of bringing services to people rather than moving people to services. For many elders, being a part of a village can delay or even prevent a move to assisted living or nursing home care.

Today there are approximately 190 villages across the country and Australia and the Netherlands with about 185 additional villages in the development stage. Most villages rely heavily on volunteers and other members to provide services and support. Villages vary depending on community needs and available resources. There are yearly fees to be a part of a village and these fees differ depending on the community and services offered.

Cohousing

Cohousing involves intentional communities that are designed to create a space where everyone has their own privacy, but shares common space. Each person or family purchases their unit or home that is linked to common space. Most cohousing communities are intergenerational and some are relegated to just older individuals. Pricing varies across the country from market rate to affordable. The design of each community reflects the shared values of its members.

Cooperatives

Cooperatives are housing communities that range from mobile home parks to high-rise apartments and single family homes. According to Beth Baker, there are approximately 6,400 nationwide. The idea is that owners have their own units or homes and share financial responsibility for common space. Cooperatives can be a very affordable option for people as they age. But keep in mind that they don't provide any of the formal supports that are offered by assisted living.

NORCs (Naturally Occurring Retirement Community)

NORCs are communities with a concentration of older people. Services are provided by agencies already working in the community that provide transportation, nursing services, educational and recreational services, and housekeeping. NORCs typically rely heavily on volunteers and their appeal is centered on the desire to remain in an already established community oftentimes years in the making.[8] NORCs were funded until 2010 by the federal government, but there is no federal funding now. It will be interesting to see how this concept can continue.

Respite Care

Respite care can refer to in-home relief for a family caregiver, but it is also an available service of many assisted living communities. The idea is simple: a furnished room in assisted living is provided for a week or two (sometimes longer) for an elder who isn't planning on living there, but needs short-term temporary care. A daily rate is paid and all of the services provided by the assisted living are afforded to the elder. An example would be that the family is leaving on an extended trip and unable or unwilling to manage in-home caregivers, so the elder lives in assisted living for the duration of the family's absence.

Another way that we have seen respite care be beneficial is for someone who is considering the move to assisted living but is uncertain if they want to commit. It can be a great opportunity to give it a try and see firsthand what living in a facility is like. One elder had been living with her daughter and her family. Her care needs were growing and her daughter had been promoted at work and could not attend to all of her mother's needs. Both the daughter and the mother considered that moving to assisted living might be the best option. But the mother was reluctant and fearful about what it would be like. The daughter and her family were going on a trip before her increased workload started and her mother decided to try out a respite stay at a nice assisted living facility nearby while they were away. She stayed there for two weeks and loved it. While there, she realized that she felt much more comfortable having a nurse on staff to help her manage her diabetes care, which was a continual worry to her. She had terrible anxiety at home wondering if she had given herself the right dose of insulin and fretted about whether she should bother her busy daughter at work. After her daughter and family returned home, they discussed it and decided that the mother would move to the assisted living facility.

PACE and LIFE Programs: Good Programs, But Not in Every State ... Yet

Medicare has had two programs for many decades that help seniors stay in their own homes and receive comprehensive, coordinated health care. One is called PACE, which stands for Programs of All-Inclusive Care for the Elderly. The other is called LIFE, which stands for Living Independence for the Elderly. Unfortunately, currently there are only thirty-six states that have either of these programs, and even in those states it is not available throughout the state. This number may be variable and likely to change.[9] To start the search to find if PACE is available to you, use the PACE plan search tool at https://www.medicare.gov/find-a-plan/questions/pace-home.aspx.

What does PACE or LIFE do? According to Medicare.gov, these programs are designed to provide a senior's healthcare needs at home instead of going to a residential care facility.[10] A PACE organization is funded with Medicare and sometimes state Medicaid dollars. They are mandated to keep the costs of one's care lower than the average cost if that person were living in nursing home care.

Traditionally, a doctor gets paid for each visit by Medicare. All doctor and other healthcare appointments (physical therapy, home health visits, hospital stays, etc.) are billed piecemeal (individual billing) to Medicare for individual visits. The care is usually not coordinated and sometimes redundant or excessive. It can also be ineffective and health issues can get worse due to neglect.

In contrast, in this model the PACE organization gets a monthly sum for each participant to provide doctor's visits, and also more services including:

- physical therapy and other rehab services
- home care
- emergency care
- prescription drugs
- adult day social and health care
- dentistry

The goal is not only to keep elders healthier and presumably happier at home, it is also to reduce the cost of nursing home care to the state and federal governments. Some participants pay a monthly fee based on their financial income and assets. Some PACE programs work in conjunction with a state Medicaid program to provide the service for no cost to the participant.

Is PACE effective? The short answer is yes. A variety of research questions have explored the outcomes of PACE programs across the country over the thirty years that it has existed. In general, the research has found that PACE and similar programs have had positive results in the following domains. A number of PACE programs have been assessed by research to find if they are more cost effective. Many studies have found that PACE programs have reduced costs to Medicare, have decreased stays in costly nursing home facilities, and have resulted in preventing and/or shortening expensive hospital stays.[11] Other research has found that PACE recipients have more comprehensive health care, better functional outcomes, and greater patient satisfaction compared to other seniors living in community.[12]

With all this good news about PACE, one wonders why it is not more accessible nationwide. Why, after being available for decades, were only forty thousand people enrolled as of January 2016 when there are millions of elderly?[13] Apparently, creating an all-encompassing, comprehensive elder care provider is no easy task. It is expensive to set up and must be accountable to the federal rules and regulations for a PACE entity. As they were originally designed, only not-for-profit organizations could start a PACE program. In a surprising and highly criticized move, the federal government decided in 2016 to open PACE to for-profit companies, hoping that this could more quickly increase its availability to more people. Elder advocates and detractors are alarmed by the prospects of yet another industry taking over and potentially reducing quality of care to a vulnerable population. As evidence of their concern, they cite uneven quality of care in the residential care sector controlled by corporations and fraud in recent decades in commercially run hospice care.[14] However, early signs show a glimmer of hope that the infusion of private sector funds could result in starting more PACE programs more quickly and provide more quality of care for a greater number of people. It will be up to oversight from the Centers for Medicare and Medicaid to ensure that this new direction is of benefit to the seniors that it is mandated to help.

WHERE THERE'S A WILL THERE'S A WAY

With motivation, imagination, and quite a bit of luck, a financial plan for good home care can be pieced together. When you work it out, it's golden. Keep in mind that while some of these suggestions might work for your family for some period of time, the elder in your life could move into a different stage that requires you to start over. Consider the following ideas.

Living with the Children, in Rotation

Here's an idea that families can do for elder care if that family has more than one adult child. After one of the grandparents has passed away, the remaining grandparent moves in with one of her children and stays for six months. Then she moves to another adult child's home for the following six months. At the end of that time, she moves back to child number one's home, and so on. Families make this work even when the move is across the state. And one family we knew had their mother move every winter from another country to stay with them. These arrangements can last several years or more depending on the health of the elder. There are many benefits. Living with the adult children can save costs and those costs can be shared by each family. The families have the experience of living multigenerationally. The closeness that evolves between grandparents and grandchildren is often a very positive gift and invaluable. Some elders might be able to provide some child care if their limitations are not too great.

One would never want the elder to feel like a hot potato or that they have to keep moving on because his or her children get tired of having them around. We've heard some elders in this situation actually express a preference to a certain adult child's home, but don't want to make waves and suggest that they stay there full time. Particular situations may arise where the moving and change might create its own problems. For instance, this strategy can make it harder for families to recognize an elder going through changes in cognition and that dementia may be developing. And someone with dementia does not usually fare well with many disruptions in their living environment.

House Sharing

As people age, it is not only access to resources and support that becomes important. Elders become widowed, children may live out of state, and it becomes impractical to stay alone in a big house with the attendant responsibilities and potential isolation that can occur. More and more people are considering house sharing as a way to pool resources and provide built-in socialization.

Some people share with a friend, and others are even willing to try sharing with strangers. The National Shared Resource Center is a clearinghouse for people who are looking to share housing and the types of arrangements people are designing are limited only by one's imagination.[15] The obvious advantages even extend to home care. If both people need help in the home, they can share in that cost.

Adult Day Services

Adult day services, sometimes referred to as adult day care, are a vital link in community-based care for older adults. Many families utilize these service centers to augment care while an elder lives with an adult child or spouse who is employed. Increasingly, elders who live alone and may have hired caregivers other hours of the day are spending more time in adult day centers.

There are many positive reasons to consider this option. [16] These adult day service centers typically provide an opportunity to increase socialization for isolated elders with activities, exercise, memory care, and field trips. Most have transportation available to and from home. They also increasingly provide more individualized and specialized care. For example, the majority of the adult day care centers offer personalized care planning, a nurse to provide medication and other doctor-ordered care, and personal care such as toileting and physical transfers from wheelchair to toilet, for example. Many have a social worker for case management. They may have physical therapy and occupational and speech therapy available at the center. Recently, more centers also provide attention to needs of specific chronic illnesses such as dementia, diabetes, and cardiovascular disease. They have special training and curriculum for memory care. They attend to foot care, monitor blood pressure and weight, and may have weight loss classes for participants. Some even offer bathing or showering if needed. And while most operate five days a week during day hours, a few are offering some hours on the weekends and even time limited twenty-four-hour care.

A longitudinal study by MetLife Mature Market Institute, the National Adult Day Center Association, and the Ohio State University College of Social Work compared the characteristics of adult day centers and their participants from 2002 to 2010. [17] Findings included:

- The number of centers across the country is growing, from 2,000 facilities in 1989 to over 4,600 in 2010.
- The average ratio of providers of hands-on care to participants is improving from 8:1 to 6:1.
- While about half of participants attend five days a week, many choose to go two to three days a week.
- The majority of participants are women over the age of sixty-five; about half have the diagnosis of dementia.
- Most adult care centers are freestanding programs, while others may be affiliated with a senior center, a nursing home, or other larger parent organization.
- Traditionally, the majority of centers have been private, not-for-profit agencies. However, there is a growing number of private, for-profit entities.

Adult day service programs can save an elder and their family money for care. A typical day is 8 a.m. to 5 p.m. and the average cost for a day at these care centers is $61.71.[18] The actual cost is closer to $68.89. As these programs usually have a variety of funding sources (state and local, fundraising, the VA, and others), they can offset the actual cost of care. Some centers charge extra for some services provided, such as for the transportation or add-on services, for instance for podiatry services. It is good to note that if an elder has long-term insurance, some of the cost of adult day services may be covered. And depending on your financial situation, you may qualify for greater assistance for the cost of care.

In short, adult day services are an important player in the endeavor to provide noninstitutional long-term care to a growing aging population. Most are striving to provide a comprehensive care model to their participants and community, very similar to those in the PACE program. While there needs to be more research, it is thought that these centers help prevent placement in nursing homes, allowing more elders to age in place. Adult day services are a sensible option for many and it is a cost effective tool for communities and states as well as for families.

The Barter System

The bartering economy is the exchange of goods or services for other goods or services and it is a system that has been around for centuries. With the increasing acceptance of the sharing economy, people are more open to consider this as a way to pay without cash for more necessary items in their life.

How does this work for caregiving? Here is an example. One caregiver we know, Angie, tells us that she enjoys having her thick long hair colored professionally and cut regularly. It is pretty pricey, but it is something that makes her happy. She has gotten to know Melinda, her stylist, well over the years. Melinda shared with Angie that her mother has Alzheimer's disease and has gotten really agitated every time Melinda tries to help her with a shower. It worries Melinda and wears her and her mother out. One day, she suggests to Angie that because she is a professional caregiver, maybe she could come and try to give Melinda's mother a shower. Angie agrees, wisely reminding Melinda that it might not work as every person with dementia is different and it could be difficult for her with a professional caregiver as well. Angie comes over and she and

Melinda's mother really hit it off; the mother simply lights up when she sees her. She really loves it when Angie comes over and the showers go smoothly. Angie says, "I like to wear sparkly earrings and her mother always notices that and I think that it cheers her up. She relaxes around me." Melinda and Angie work out a system that Angie will get her long tresses cut and colored regularly once a month and Angie comes over six times a month to give Melinda's mother a shower.

In fact, this kind of informal trade for service is not unheard of and has been going on for some time. Some caregivers provide a certain number of hours of care to an elder in exchange for car repair. Others trade elder care for child care. A key component seems to be that the two parties involved know each other through previous experience.

A caveat: bartering is legal as long as taxes are paid.[19] For example, if you trade $200 dollars' worth of caregiving service for $200 dollars' worth of hair salon service, both professionals must document and pay the taxes for that service on the Form 1040. If taxes are not paid, this would be considered "under the table" and is illegal. Consult with your accountant or attorney to make sure that you are following the law.

More commonly, there are those that exchange with someone, usually a young person, room and board for being a live-in caregiver. We recently heard of a family who had a very bad experience with poor quality care from an agency. The agency sent a different caregiver every week. The caregivers who arrived would not do much more than sit around and did not even prepare an evening meal for the elder. The family and the elder were outraged by this and unhappy at the high cost. In response, they decided to find someone to exchange room and board for being in the home with the elder at night and find someone else for shorter day hours. They expect that this will not only meet the needs of the elder involved more effectively, but also cost less. This family also needs to consult their attorney or accountant to make sure that the value of the room and board is legally documented for both parties and that any taxes accrued are paid. Bartering may offer an opportunity for people to exchange services and skills in a creative way that improves the care of elders.

Home Improvements for Savings: From Basics to Universal Design

You may not think of spending money on home improvements as a cost saver, but there may be some financial benefits in certain situations. When an elder or a family takes the initiative to make an existing home more accessible by adding grab bars in the bathroom or building a ramp to the entry for a wheelchair to have access, they are decreasing the likelihood or at least delaying that the elder will be placed in a nursing home. States, through the Medicaid program, are the major payers for nursing home care. Consequently, some states are beginning to realize that they can reduce high Medicaid costs by providing state tax credits to their citizens who make these types of home improvements.[20] For example, Virginia has the Virginia Livable Home Tax Credit. People of all ages who do work on an existing home to improve accessibility can get up to $5,000 in credits. And if they are purchasing a new, more accessible home, they can also get up to $5,000 in tax credit. There are counties in other states that have similar credits and legislation is being considered to follow suit in a number of states. This effort is supported by disability advocates as well as real estate businesses as it can enhance the value of the home.

In addition, there are great strides in "universal design" or housing that is designed to be accessible for all abilities at any age. There is no need to retrofit this type of home as it is designed to adapt to the lifetime of the inhabitants.[21] The concept informs the construction of the entire home. The doorways are widened to accommodate a wheelchair or stroller. There is at least one entrance that is accessible without stairs. Door handles, rather than slippery door knobs, are the norm. The great thing is that these homes do not necessarily look different than any other home. They simply have greater ease of use for a wider variety of people.

One might assume that these homes are all very expensive and certainly some may be. However, just as states are seeing an opportunity to reduce Medicaid costs by offering tax credits to retrofit older houses, some locales are also providing tax credits toward the purchase of these smart constructions. And some areas (parts of Arizona and Illinois) are changing zoning laws to encourage universal design and even making it mandatory.[22]

PAYINGFORSENIORCARE.COM: ONLINE TOOLS TO CONNECT YOUR FAMILY TO RESOURCES

We spoke with Alex Guerrero, the director of operations of the American Elder Care Research Organization, which manages the website Payingforseniorcare.com. This website is one that we have perused many times in the course of researching this chapter. There is an abundance of ideas to find ways to pay for senior care. Importantly, the site offers online tools to connect elders and their families to specific programs to find out if their particular situation qualifies for a certain resource. Here is some of the discussion that we had with Alex.

The website Payingforseniorcare.com has been up since 2008. What are some of the trends that you have noticed since starting the website?

The traffic on the site has gone up and up. We find that there is a seasonality to the traffic. There is a big lull at the holidays, December is very, very slow, and then it increases again in January and February.

We've discovered that families are in different stages: some are just at the diagnosis point, say with Alzheimer's and starting to look, or they are in a crisis like "How are we going to pay?" They are coming at it from completely different angles. We try and accommodate for whatever the mindset the family has.

A lot of voicemails and e-mails have more detailed questions. "Thank you for providing this information, I'm still overwhelmed." "Can you help me get to the next level with a financial plan?" "I'm so busy being the caregiver that I can't simultaneously figure out a financial plan. I need more help." We try to look at this from a technology perspective. How can we help people by applying technology to the problem? And so we have built several interactive tools that help people further along that process. There is a limit of what we can do from a technology perspective and a resource perspective.

We look at the financial side of paying for home care as a two-stage process: there is discovery or defining a need and discovery of what the options are. "Now I know my options, how do I put these puzzle pieces together?" We help families on the discovery side.

For example, you are trying to care for a parent at home who is wheelchair bound. They might need a caregiver and they may need some home modifications and they might live in a rural area of the country. Most people would never think to go to the USDA as a financial source. It wouldn't occur to people to go to the Department of Agriculture. Yet the USDA has a program that helps low-income elderly residents in rural areas remain living in their homes. They do not have to be a farmer. There is really obscure stuff out there. We help with that discovery side. Tell us your situation. We have all that in the database. We're not going to tell you the programs that you are eligible for because that's very limiting. But we tell you the programs that are relevant to your situation, which are a broader set of programs. The situations are always changing. You may be very soon eligible for program x, y, or z.

We spend a large percentage of our time digging around and looking for the possibilities and another large percent of our time making sure that the information is current. So once a year we rewrite the entire website. These programs are constantly changing and the eligibility requirements are constantly changing. Some programs expire. So it takes a major effort, but if we weren't to do that the information would become dated very quickly.

What are some of the most creative ways that you have heard of people doing to pay for senior care?

At least twenty times a day, we get asked, "Can I get paid as a caregiver for my loved one?" One of the more creative solutions that I've heard of is that in certain states, California being one of them, also Rhode Island and New Jersey, they have a version of the federal family medical leave act, which will pay a family member a percentage of their salary if they have to take time off to care for a loved one. Most have been designed for new parents, but they have been broadened to take care of aging parents. Most are designed for you to take six weeks off and they'll hold your job. But those six weeks do not need to be consecutive. You can take one day off a week for forty-two weeks a year, which is essentially the whole year. DC is working on it and New York may have it in 2018.

SHOUT OUT TO CAREGIVERS

A big part of the puzzle in making home care work is the availability of good caregivers. As we look at creative solutions for making home care accessible to all, it appears that the home care industry must reshape itself to address the realities of both clients and staff. Many savvy home care administrators are already recognizing that the industry must learn more about their employees, their lives, and their challenges in order to build and retain the best quality workforce.

As we have mentioned, caregivers are some of the lowest paid workers in America with an annual medium income of $13,300.[23] Twenty-four percent of home care workers live in households below the federal poverty line. And the demand for these workers will continue to grow with the home care occupation expected to add more jobs than any other occupation. As the nationwide effort to increase the minimum wage to $15 an hour gains steam, there is hope among home care workers that their income will increase. Consumers rightly expect that care staff are competent, trained, and professional. The home care industry bears some of the responsibility in assuring that this happens, and many are leading the effort to recruit and retain good, qualified staff.

As an owner of a private duty care agency said to us, "our caregivers lead complicated lives." That is probably an understatement. Somehow these caring and dedicated professionals find a way to do the work they love while often struggling to make ends meet. Agencies and online companies are beginning to recognize that they have a responsibility to their caregivers to be a part of the solution in providing a living wage and other benefits to their employees. Recruiting and retaining staff has become more challenging than ever, with home health companies, nursing homes, and assisted living communities all competing for the same qualified caregivers. Here are some ways in which agencies and online companies have added value to what they offer their employees:

- One owner told us that she offers "loans" to her employees during emergencies. The amount is taken out of the next paycheck. She states: "Employers need to be more flexible in this industry. I do what is necessary to keep my caregivers staying with me, even if it means doing things outside what would be considered customary practices for an employer."

- Another small agency owner has an extra car. She has loaned it to caregivers who are in a jam with their own vehicle or transportation. The owner recognizes that an important part of her company's reputation is that caregivers show up to work on time. Having this car available when a caregiver is in need makes a difference for the caregiver to be able to keep her shift and for the company to uphold quality standards.

- Bonuses: many of the agency owners we spoke with offer bonuses like gift cards or gas cards to employees who do exceptional work.

- Provide recognition: The best agencies give regular verbal recognition to their best caregivers.

- Regular training helps caregivers feel more confident in the work they are doing. Training adds a layer of professionalism and a stake in the company.

- Flexible scheduling: Scheduling is the most complex part of what an agency does, but meeting a caregiver's needs with regard to scheduling can go a long way to keeping them satisfied in the job.

- Paying for additional professional training: Some companies are offering to pay an employee to become a Certified Nursing Assistant, which often translates to higher pay.

- Online companies are beginning to make inroads into adding value to their business by making their caregivers employees, offering paid sick leave, stock options, increased training, and career advancement opportunities. [24]

- Another model that has been established in various parts of the country is that of the workers' cooperative. As described by Ai-Jen Poo in her book *The Age of Dignity: Preparing for the Elder Boom in a Changing America*, home care cooperatives are home care worker-owned and feature "full-time hours, competitive wages, overtime paid at time-and-a-half of base wage, worker ownership, peer mentoring, financial literacy training, and supervision that balances coaching, support, and accountability. As a result, their annual turnover rate is half the industry average."[25]

SUMMARY

In all of the alternatives we have discussed in this chapter, the bottom line is that elders and families can find a wide variety of options for aging in place, senior housing, and paying for care. Seniors should never be kept in isolation. They benefit, as we all do, in numerous ways from community contact, support, and engagement in decisions that affect their lives.

TAKEAWAY POINTS FOR THIS CHAPTER

- When making a financial plan for aging in place and home care, consider all the different programs and possibilities that can be part of the creative solution for your elder.
- Some programs can assist in the care of an elder living at home. Some require that the elder move to another home rather than a larger facility. Weigh the pros and cons of such a choice.
- Find out if comprehensive care programs, such as PACE and LIFE, are in place in your community. These programs can be a great benefit in that they consider all of the person's care as a whole, eliminating overlap and providing better quality of care.
- Consider adult day services and other programs and traditional practices such as barter and trade for care that may ease the financial cost of staying at home.
- Use online tools such as on payingforseniorcare.com to find resources and possibilities to assist with the cost of care.
- When hiring a care agency, find out how they treat their employees. When professional caregivers are treated with respect, the client usually benefits.

10

COMING HOME

INTRODUCTION

We began this book with the story of Leslie's discovery of theft and the exploitation of her elder parents by a trusted caregiver. In this chapter, we will tell you the rest of the tale and how Leslie and her family had to adapt to a new reality. She will share what it has been like for her personally to go through this nightmarish situation, regroup, and rethink her approach. She will share the process of making a decision to try a home care agency instead of hiring caregivers privately. Finally, both Leslie and Amanda will discuss what they have learned in the process of writing about hiring caregivers.

Leslie's Story

As you may recall from the beginning of the book, I called and fired Marsha the caregiver when my suspicions were confirmed that she was charging personal items on my parents' credit card. When she heard that she was being fired, Marsha actually asked if there was a warrant out for her arrest. It was clear that there was more criminal activity to uncover.

I started by calling the police and filing a report of missing jewelry and credit card fraud. Before the case was assigned to a detective, I called Adult Protective Services. Unfortunately, I learned that since I had already fired the caregiver, APS could not come assess the situation. They could only investigate if the alleged exploitation was still occurring. The

APS caseworker did offer suggestions and support on how to proceed. I learned that even if Marsha was convicted, my parents' state does not keep a list of offenders who exploit the elderly. The only way that APS in that state could forewarn a potential employer is if the convicted person was licensed and had that license removed due to a criminal record. In this particular case, the caregiver was not licensed.

I met with the police detective to go over the details of the report. As it happened, the prosecuting attorney was in the police station that day reviewing cases. The prosecuting attorney and the detective were very helpful in directing me to look for particular kinds of evidence that could be used to convict. Sadly, they had many stories of financial abuse and exploitation of other older people in the area. As we have discussed in a previous chapter, many elders and their families are reluctant to follow through with the legal process to convict. It can be a long ordeal itself and an ongoing reminder of being violated. In the cases of stolen jewelry or material possessions, the case can be hard to try. It can be difficult to find stolen jewelry. It can devolve into one person's word against another. Prosecutors with huge caseloads are wary of taking on cases they don't think they can win. Without hard and fast evidence, many of these cases are let go.

I talked with my parents and my sister. We had all not only liked Marsha, but also felt that she had become like a member of the family. Even though my parents were confused about how such a nice person whom we had all grown to trust could steal from them, they were also embarrassed that they could have let it happen to them. My sister and I felt the same way and both of us felt deeply violated. I told my family how sorry I was that I had let this person into their home and their life. I was angry at the thief and with myself for not knowing what was going on. We all agreed on one thing: this person did something criminal and should go to jail. As a family, we made the decision to proceed with the police case.

As with any crisis situation, many things were happening at once. First and foremost, I needed to make sure that my parents were secure and well taken care of by trusted caregivers. Fortunately, I have a lifelong friend, Sarah, who had started a small but reliable home care company. She had already been providing fill-ins from time to time when another caregiver was off. Sarah was more than happy to help out and provided staffing while I started a search for a replacement. Even though I was going through this terrible situation related to hiring privately, I still wanted to do that rather than have a long-term plan with an agency. By then I had learned that the caregiver whom we had trusted had a criminal drug history. As you can imagine, the search for a new caregiver had a whole new set of criteria: background checks, drug screening, and more intensive scrutiny.

In addition, home security became paramount. Locks, credit cards, and bank accounts were changed. The house was searched for missing valuables, mail, receipts, and any clues of further theft. There were frustrating turns and twists. It was too easy to speculate about bad things that Marsha did or might have done. There were lots of sleepless nights, self-blame, and so many thoughts of "why didn't I figure this out sooner?" Efforts to help the police investigation for solid evidence were like searching for a needle in a haystack.

Then a lucky piece of mail arrived. As power of attorney, I had changed the mailing address for any sensitive mail to come to my address in another state. However, some had continued to come to my parents' address without my knowledge. A check arrived in the mail, leading me to wonder if previous checks had been sent. I contacted the company that had sent the check. It turned out that a number of other checks had been sent during the time that Marsha had worked at my parents' home. She had had my parents sign over the checks to her, telling them that she would deposit them in their bank account. Marsha then deposited all the checks into her own bank account. The police were able to follow and obtain documents from this paper trail for actual proof of illegal activity.

While we may assume that legal cases and crimes are solved quickly the way they are on TV and the movies, they are not. After the initial arrest, the caregiver in question got out on bond and we soon learned that Marsha was again working as a caregiver for another elderly person. Until convicted, there was nothing that could be done to stop this. My sister and I were very upset. We feared for the safety and security of this other family.

Marsha's defense attorney sent large envelopes addressed to my parents filled with lengthy letters implying that their honesty and reputation would be on trial in the courtroom and other intimidation tactics. The prosecuting attorney assured me that these efforts were "mere puffery," but it was discouraging as intended. There were delays and court dates were rescheduled. Finally, over a year later, the case was heard in court and the caregiver was convicted. At the sentencing, the judge told Marsha that she would go to jail and on release would never be allowed to work in any setting as a caregiver for an elder or vulnerable adult again.

THE CAREGIVING JOURNEY CONTINUES

After that harrowing experience, I continued to hire caregivers privately for my parents. I believed, as I still do, that the criminal caregiver was the exception. As my parents had twenty-four-hour care, I still had a couple of good, honest, and skilled caregivers on board. I knew that I could find good people and save my parents' money by doing the hiring myself. I was determined to rebuild the team to make it better and stronger.

It helps that I became more than a little obsessive about it. I was determined not to let a crook ruin my parents' goal to stay at home. I set up interviews with caregivers that I found online and by word of mouth. I arranged to meet each caregiver on a video call. I asked for input from my sister and my parents when possible. However, my parents could find something wrong with even the best candidate. Finally, I had to say that I would take their input seriously, but that I would make the final hiring decision.

As with any workforce, some terrific caregivers move, finish school, or go to another job with more hours, and I have had to repeat the hiring process over and over. Now I explain to each potential job candidate that there will be a background check and drug screening. At first, this was not comfortable for me to do. I was apprehensive about how people would react. For the most part, I have been relieved that the response to that information has largely been solid agreement. In fact, a number of people, when I tell them that I will run a background check, have said, "Of course, you are very smart to do that. I would do that too if someone was taking care of my mother. There are a lot of bad people out there!" If I note any hesitation or negativity about that requirement, I know that it is time to move on to the next applicant. I will admit that there have been times when there was great pressure to quickly hire someone and to skip the time-consuming steps of vetting the caregiver. For me, it is an understatement to say that it is hard to be many states away and hire a caregiver to fill such an important role in my parents' lives. When I have felt the constraint of time, however, I would be reminded of that haunting feeling of my parents being victimized.

A PERSONAL PERSPECTIVE: PRIVATE HIRE VERSUS CARE AGENCY

Eventually, things were sorted out and we resumed life with caregivers for my parents. We developed a team of people who were caring, loyal, and reliable. I continued in my role as the employer and manager of the caregivers and my parents' care for another couple of years.

My parents had some difficult chronic illnesses that were progressing. The care became more challenging. There were more urgent calls, trips to the ER, and complications to be dealt with. With each visit with them, I could see changes in my parents' health. I had a growing awareness that my time with my parents was becoming limited. It became evident that I was spending a great deal of time managing the schedule, payroll, and taxes, ordering supplies, and trying to settle disagreements between care-givers about how things should be done. There were so many details. I came to the realization that I was spending more time on those parts of my being a family member than actually speaking and spending time with my parents.

Much of this happened during the writing of this book. I had begun to wonder if Amanda's approach in only hiring through a home care agency might relieve me of some of my responsibilities so that I could focus more on the time I had with my parents. I considered that maybe it was time to hand over the reins to a home care agency. As it happened, on one of my visits to my parents, I heard about an agency in their area that appeared to have a more forward thinking approach to their caregiver employees than others in the area and had a reputation of high respon-siveness to client needs. They also had a nurse supervisor, a role that is critical in caring for people with more complex medical issues. They paid their employees a fair salary, provided good training, and offered more flexible schedules. I called them to learn about their story as part of the research for this book. Months later, I decided to arrange for them to take on the home care of my parents. Some of our privately hired caregivers, with some skepticism about working for any agency and a great deal of love and loyalty to my parents, agreed to the offer from the agency to work for them so that they could continue to assist my parents.

With this transition, I have been relieved of my duties as the employee manager and the huge time requirement for searching for applicants, hiring, firing, scheduling, and payroll. I am able to spend more time talking with my parents. However, some aspects of being the family care manager have not changed. There are still so many components and minutiae of my parents' care to contend with. I have been learning firsthand what the advantages and disadvantages are to both choices. Below is an update of my own personal list of pros and cons.

Leslie's pros of a home care agency:

- It is a great relief for someone else to do the due diligence required for the background screening of prospective employees. It is time consuming and requires a great deal of objectivity. When you have asked as many questions as I have about the hiring process of an agency and the answers are good, it is great to let someone else be in charge of that job.
- I appreciate the nurse supervisor. In fact, I would not have decided to make this transition if I had not had the chance to talk with this vital team member beforehand. The particular agency that we have hired has a tremendously skilled and experienced nurse at the helm of clinical care. She has patiently gone through minute details of my parents' complicated care (over and over) to develop the care plan. She updates it as needed and has responded to multiple e-mails and phone calls to clarify and modify at my request.
- I like being able to see the schedule of who is on and make requests to change if someone is not a good fit. Before, if a caregiver and my parent were not a good fit, it would not necessarily be something easy to change. After all, I had already gone through the time and energy to seek and hire them. We had made a commitment to them as they had to us. With an agency, however, we could face the reality that it just isn't working as well as it could with a different person and request that change. The scheduler is very helpful and can tell me more about each caregiver if I have questions or requests.

- I am so glad that I do not have to find a fill-in if the caregiver is sick that day. The agency has people to be the backup and that lifts a burden from my shoulders.

Leslie's cons of a home care agency:

- The cost is much higher. I put off this transition as long as possible, but at least I now have a clear view of the financial value of what I had been doing for years. I can see the amount of money that we saved by my doing the employee management for as long as I did.
- The state laws restricting what an agency home caregiver cannot do for clients continue to astound me, even though I was expecting some. Can't fill the medication box. Can't crush pills needed for someone who has difficulty swallowing. Can't give liquid medication unless it has been premeasured. Can't give acetaminophen "as needed" for pain, only a standing, 'round-the-clock order. Can't trim fingernails even with a safety clipper. Can't change even a simple dressing that is really not different from a large Band-Aid. Unfortunately for our family, these realities came at a time when we needed these simple tasks done every day. We had to scramble to figure out an alternative. My sister was able to come do extra tasks very early before going to work and most days she also had to come in the evening. This had never been a problem with the privately hired caregivers. With our permission and their agreement, they could do whatever task we requested. As a former home health nurse, I had taught many family members in the home to do these same simple jobs for another family member. We routinely taught these simple care assignments and more complex ones such as wound care and dressing changes and drawing up a dose of insulin and using a syringe to give required medications ordered by a physician. None of these family members were licensed and all had varied levels of education. Yet they were perfectly capable of doing these tasks correctly. The laws governing home care staff evolve from regulations covering Certified Nurse Assistants working in a nursing home or other residential or institutional setting. However, limiting a home caregiver with those same set of standards doesn't make sense. It makes aging at home much more costly and complicated than it needs to be.

- While there have been some really fantastic caregivers through the agency, it took months to attain consistently scheduled people. They may have other jobs or classes to attend. Some really good caregivers simply did not want to work with someone who had complicated care or needed help with transfers. Over the first few months of agency care, my parents had too many different caregivers. Some they would only see for one shift and never again. Others were filling in during their school break and then had to return to school. With our privately hired caregivers, people wanted consistent shifts and stuck with them for years. My parents had the same person that they knew they could count on. Over time, we finally have a more reliable and consistent team of caregivers, but it has taken patience and a long time to get there.
- Communication can be difficult. It has taken me a while to get used to not being able communicate with each caregiver by e-mail or text when something comes up as I had previously with the privately hired team. I could send out a simple group e-mail, such as "Please have my mother drink extra fluid on Tuesday morning before the home health nurse comes by to draw blood." Now I send that message to the scheduler at the agency, but it is clear that not all the caregivers get the message. The agency discourages employees from contacting me. Fortunately, we have a "house" cell phone and I encourage caregivers to use it to keep me posted by text to let me know if there are concerns that I need to know about. Living in a different time zone makes it a challenge to make phone calls for every item, so texting is a quick and convenient method of communication. I have recently learned that our agency is getting a new online software that will allow families greater access to sending group messages to all of the caregivers.

THE INVISIBLE COSTS OF BEING THE FAMILY CARE MANAGER

There is no doubt that traditional family caregivers who provide the actual 'round-the-clock care to their loved one in the home suffer from a great deal of stress. They not only do the physical care, they are also often unable to leave their family member in another person's care. In my mental health practice, I have frequently seen spouses, usually wives, who had cared for a partner with chronic illnesses such as diabetes, heart disease, and dementia in their home for many years. It had not only taken a physical toll on their own health, but also impacted their overall mental well-being. They frequently had problems with depression and anxiety related to the huge workload that they had endured. The care has an emotional cost.

Even when you are not the hands-on caregiver in a family but bear the responsibility of managing that care, you can endure a lot of stress that have emotional consequences. Every situation is different. However, whether you live close by your elder family member with a professional caregiver or across the country, you may relate to some of the concerns that I have faced:

- Decision fatigue: You may have noticed reading this chapter that I like to have a lot of control! However, the day in and day out oversight of my parents' care can lead to what I think of as "decision fatigue." I am just plain tired of being the one to decide so many issues.

- The dreaded middle of the night phone call: I have had many of these calls over the years while my parents have been aging at home with caregivers. They are usually due to a medical crisis that requires a decision about whether or not to go to the ER and for me to coordinate how that is going to occur. When we had privately hired caregivers, it could be that someone's child was sick and they wouldn't be able to come for their shift at 7 a.m., requiring that I start calling and e-mailing to see if we could get quick coverage. I will admit that I have occasionally woken up from a deep sleep having imagined the phone ringing in the middle of the night to find that it hasn't.

- Fear of forgetting some critical detail: There are only so many details that you can handle in one day. Between raising my own children and my daily work and responsibilities, I also have what I term my "virtual life." I am aware of my parents' lives by phone, by e-mail, by text, by security cameras, and by video call. I get information from my parents and family and the caregivers, as well as from their doctors, the physical therapist, and the home health nurse. At times it is minute by minute. I can be driving in the town where I live many miles from them and I am getting calls and trying to solve problems far, far away. I pick my kids up from school and as they get in the car, I am holding up my hand to indicate that they need to be quiet while I am on the phone dealing with issues about their grandparents' care. They know the drill and wait until I am off the phone to tell me about their day.

- Energy depletion: There are times in the cycles of care that I would feel actually energized by a crisis or a sudden issue for my parents or their care. As a nurse and a social worker, I am keen to find the parts of the puzzle to solve a problem. How can I find wheelchair transportation in my parents' small town? Can the doctor order the hospital bed before my parent is discharged from the hospital? Should we get a second opinion about the diagnosis and treatment? At other times, after a number of years of this, I just didn't think that I could manage it all anymore. It had all seemed doable at an earlier point. But as my parents' health worsened, it got harder for me to maintain the energy for the 24/7, week after week, month after month oversight of care. This is different from what I described earlier as decision fatigue. In other words, I was physically and emotionally exhausted too. It does not necessarily get easier with the passing of time.

IF I HAD TO DO IT OVER AGAIN, WHAT WOULD I DO DIFFERENTLY?

In terms of the hiring of caregivers, I think that if I had to do it over again, I would again hire privately, but with more fastidious attention to security and background screening. I would have continued to do it that way rather than with a care agency. All of this is extremely expensive. It was less costly when we hired privately. However, if I was starting over and knew more, as I do now, about building in protections for security and the skill of the caregivers, I think that I would have done a better job overall. And with hindsight I would probably have sought out a good geriatric care manager to share the oversight of care with me. I would have to find one who would be willing to accept that our caregivers were privately hired and not agency staff. I think if I had done that from the beginning, I probably would not have felt the need to move on to working with a care agency.

For all of the above, I have had to look at my need for control with some self-reflection and self-compassion. A couple of years into this and after the criminal caregiver, I would feel very guilty that I had made so many errors and not taken better care of my parents. Eventually, I let myself off the hook. Yes, I have made just about every mistake that we warn you against in the earlier chapters. At the end of the day, I am just as human as anyone else.

I do the best that I can, but I have learned that I cannot control the universe. My parents have been grateful for most of my efforts to help them. (Except for taking away the car—I don't know if I will ever be forgiven for that.) My mantra has become "it is what it is."

Amanda's Journey

It seems as if not a day goes by that in casual conversation, at parties, at the gym, or with friends and acquaintances the conversation turns to care of parents and grandparents. Each story is unique and choices are made because they must be made—sometimes very quickly and sometimes with virtually no knowledge, and other times, though rarely, with a good solid idea of how the healthcare system works.

As Leslie and I have written this book, I too have had my own rather fixed notions of how elder care should be handled turned upside down. The most basic lesson I have learned is that there is no "right" or "correct" way for everyone. However, having knowledge allows us and our elders to make informed choices about what is right for the moment. That moment will pass and change, allowing for more decisions.

As a professional care manager, I do not recommend that families look outside licensed agencies for care. I depend on a company's background checks, liability insurance, and payment of employee taxes. However, as a consumer I would do what I need to do to provide care for my own parents.

My friend Cindy, whose mom lives across the country in a different state, recently told me a story that perfectly describes how decisions get made. Her mom was hospitalized with an exacerbation of her congestive heart failure. She was already struggling to live independently and now she was in a more weakened state and needed help at home. With virtually no notice, she was told she was being discharged from the hospital with no one available to take care of her. The family gathered in the hospital to discuss what to do and a nurse overheard the discussion. She told the family that there was a group of women who provide home care "under the table." Cindy's mom had long-term care insurance, but the waiting period was one hundred days. The family contacted one of these women to stay with their mom twenty-four hours a day at $7.00 an hour. I was aghast at the price of $7.00 an hour. I asked if she was concerned about the risks of hiring someone she doesn't know, and she said yes, she was, but that they were desperate to find someone until they could use an agency through the long-term care insurance. They also knew that it could take a care agency a couple of days or longer to staff the care that their mom needed and they couldn't wait.

Would I have made the same decision? I may have. But I probably would have worked to get the care staffed through a reputable agency if I had the financial resources to do so and could find an agency that I trusted. $168 for a twenty-four-hour period at $7.00 an hour is much different than the going rate of $20 an hour with an agency bringing the total to $480 for a twenty-four-hour period. I would be suspect of someone willing to work for this little per hour, but desperate times sometimes call for desperate measures. My friend rationalized her decision by saying that the family would eventually go through an agency. It is a risk they were willing to take.

Most people come to these very personal decisions with a measure of naivety because, like most unpleasant experiences in life, they prefer to deal with the problem when it arises. The majority of calls I get either from friends and family or as a professional are almost always panicked. The anxiety people feel at not understanding how our healthcare system works and what resources are available for people as they age is completely understandable. When you have twenty-four hours to make a decision it can be tough to get up to speed on everything you need to know!

How has my thinking changed? Over the years I have observed a slow change in the agencies that I hire as a professional. On the one hand, some are outstanding. But as more and more people jump into the industry and begin vying for the same care staff, it can be a real challenge to find committed, qualified, and responsible staff. The competition may be good in that it forces companies to perform better, but some agencies seem to be in it just for what they see as a profit-making venture.

The time it takes to manage and monitor the care staff of an agency is significant. The critical challenge to hiring through an agency is communication. The additional layer of communication that an agency requires is the most frustrating and potentially problematic aspect of this choice. Most agencies do not allow a consumer to talk directly to a care provider regarding changes in care, problems, or other issues (which is understandable). Every agency has its method of communication: family portals, care journals at the home, or a care manager to talk to at the agency. All of these methods have problems. Being able to talk directly to a caregiver that I hire has significant appeal and might tip me in the direction of hiring outside an agency.

The other appeal of hiring outside an agency is being able to choose the caregiver myself to fit the needs of my family member. With an agency I know only too well how hard they try to find a good fit, but many times a decision is made based on availability. I like the idea of choosing the care provider myself. The bottom line is that I would most likely start with an agency, but would be more willing now to look at other options if I could not find an agency to meet my elder's needs.

SUMMARY

During the writing of this book, many issues regarding hiring caregivers for home care have been evolving almost as quickly as the aging demographic is growing. For example, the laws governing overtime pay have been established by the federal government to include home care agency staff. The law was then challenged by Congress and frozen. Then it was unfrozen and put into practice. Now these laws may be up for grabs again in the future.

We read on an almost daily basis of changes in the home care industry. There is new technology for security and software designed to enhance aging and home caregiving. There are new trends in how and who to hire for these critical roles.

We are excited to see the new patterns and expectations that the baby boomers are instituting for their advancing age. We think that many good things will come of their pioneering spirit in shaping and controlling their own terms for aging. As their demands for a good quality of life continue, it will influence the way that home care is delivered across the country.

We hope this book has informed, educated, and prepared the reader to face the challenges of aging with care at home with confidence and calm.

GLOSSARY OF TERMS

Activities of Daily Living (ADLs): Routine activities that people tend to do every day without needing assistance. There are six basic ADLs: eating, bathing, dressing, toileting, walking, and transferring oneself from bed or chair to standing and continence.

Adult Protective Services (APS) : Adult Protective Services is a social services program provided by state and local governments nationwide serving seniors and adults with disabilities who are in need of assistance. APS workers frequently serve as first responders in cases of abuse, neglect, or exploitation, working closely with a wide variety of allied professionals such as physicians, nurses, paramedics, firefighters, and law enforcement officers.

Advance Directives : An advance healthcare directive and durable power of attorney for health care can also be known as a living will, personal directive, advance directive, medical directive, or advance decision. It is a legal document in which a person specifies what actions should be taken for their health if they are no longer able to make decisions for themselves because of illness or incapacity.

Alzheimer's Association: The Alzheimer's Association works on a global, national, and local level to enhance care and support for all those affected by Alzheimer's and other dementias.

Assisted Living : A system of housing and limited care that is designed for senior citizens who need some assistance with daily activities but do not require care in a nursing home.

Certified Nursing Assistant (CNA): A licensed caregiver who has had designated training to care for adults under the supervision of a nurse with daily living needs such as bathing, dressing, using the toilet, assisting with transfers from a bed to a chair, meal preparation, eating assistance, and handing/cueing medication on schedule. Each state's Board of Nursing determines the number of hours of training and licensing.

Dementia: A general term for a decline in mental ability severe enough to interfere with daily life. Memory loss is an example. Alzheimer's is the most common type of dementia.

Dignity of Risk: Respecting each individual's autonomy and self-determination (or "dignity") to make choices for him- or herself. The concept means that all adults have the right to make their own choices about their health and care, even if healthcare professionals believe these choices endanger the person's health or longevity.

Emergency Response System (ERS): A medical alarm is an alarm system designed to signal the presence of a hazard requiring urgent attention and to summon emergency medical personnel. Other terms for a medical alarm are personal emergency response system (PERS) or medical alert.

Estate Planning: The act of preparing for the transfer of a person's wealth and assets after his or her death. Assets, life insurance, pensions, real estate, cars, personal belongings, and debts are all part of one's estate. Estate planning may also involve developing advanced directives.

Geriatric Care Manager or Aging Life Care Professional: An Aging Life Care Professional, also known as a geriatric care manager, is a health and human services specialist who acts as a guide and advocate for families who are caring for older relatives or disabled adults. The Aging Life Care Professional is educated and experienced in any of several fields related to aging life care/care management, including but not limited to nursing, gerontology, social work, or psychology, with a specialized focus on issues related to aging and elder care.

Guardianship: A legal relationship created when a person or institution is named in a will or assigned by the court to take care of minor children or incompetent adults. Sometimes called a conservatorship.

Health Care Assistant (HCA): Clinical support staff who work under a licensed healthcare provider. While this generally occurs in a professional setting such as a nursing home or assisted living, some HCAs become home caregivers.

HIPAA: HIPAA is the Health Insurance and Portability and Accountability Act. It is legislation that provides data privacy and security provisions for safeguarding medical information.

Home Health Aide (HHA): Home health aides help people with disabilities, chronic illness, or cognitive impairment with activities of daily living. They often help older adults who need assistance. In some states, home health aides may be able to give a client medication or check the client's vital signs under the direction of a nurse or other healthcare practitioner.

Home Health Care: Home health care is a service ordered by a doctor for brief, time-limited home visits by a Registered Nurse, physical therapist, occupational therapist, speech therapist, or home health aide. Home health care is typically paid for by Medicare or other medical insurance programs. It is different from nonmedical care such as home care provided by a caregiver hired privately or through an agency.

Medicaid: A healthcare program that assists low-income families or individuals in paying for long-term medical and custodial care costs. Medicaid is a joint program funded primarily by the federal government and run at the state level, where coverage may vary.

Medicare: A federal health insurance program for people who are sixty-five or older, certain younger people with disabilities, and people with end-stage renal disease (permanent kidney failure requiring dialysis or a transplant, sometimes called ESRD).

Memory Care Unit: Typically found in assisted living communities. A residential area devoted to people who have dementia or other cognitive impairment issues.

Nursing Home: A public or private residential facility providing a high level of long-term personal and nursing care for persons (such as the aged or the chronically ill) who are unable to care for themselves properly.

Personal Care: Another name for private duty care.

Private Duty Care: Private duty care is a service provided to elderly individuals who are in need of assistance with day-to-day activities. A private duty home caregiver visits your home or the home of your loved one and helps with activities such as meal preparation, housekeeping, and personal grooming and hygiene. Typically, these services are private pay.

Rehabilitation Care Facility: An inpatient rehabilitation facility is a facility licensed under state laws to provide skilled nursing care and intensive rehabilitative services.

Respite Care: Temporary institutional care of a dependent elderly, ill, or handicapped person, providing relief for their usual caregivers.

Supported Decision Making: An alternative to guardianship that allows an individual with a disability to work with a team and make his or her own choices about his or her own life. Under this model, the individual designates people to be part of a support network to help with decision making. Supported decision making promotes self-determination, control, and autonomy. It fosters independence. Unlike *substituted* decision making, in which guardians, family members, or caregivers make decisions for the individual, *supported* decision making enables the person to make his or her own decisions with assistance from a trusted network of supporters.

Transfers: Refers to the physical assistance by a caregiver to help a person move from one place to another, such as from the bed to a chair or a wheelchair to a toilet. Some people can be transferred by one person and others require a two-person assist or a transfer device such as a Hoyer lift.

Waiver Programs: Within broad federal guidelines, states can develop home- and community-based services waivers (HCBS waivers) to meet the needs of people who prefer to get long-term care services and supports in their home or community rather than in an institutional setting. In 2009, nearly one million individuals were receiving services under HCBS waivers. Nearly all states plus Washington, DC, offer services through HCBS waivers. States can operate as many HCBS waivers as they want—currently, more than three hundred HCBS waiver programs are active nationwide.

NOTES

1. TWO APPROACHES TO HIRING CAREGIVERS

1. AARP Public Policy Institute, "Aging in Place. A State Survey of Livability Policies and Practices," a Research Report by the National Conference of State Legislatures and the AARP Public Policy Institute, accessed December 2, 2016, http://assets.aarp.org/rgcenter/ppi/liv-com/ib190.pdf.

2. U.S. Census Bureau, "Census Shows 65 and Older Population Growing Faster than Total U.S. Population," accessed December 2, 2016, https://www.census.gov/newsroom/releases/archives/2010_census/cb11-cn192.html.

3. Paraprofessional Healthcare Institute, "Report on How Poverty Wages Undermine Care," accessed December 2, 2016, http://phinational.org/research-reports/paying-price-how-poverty-wages-undermine-home-care-americastititue.

4. Ibid.

5. Jane Brody, "Staying Independent in Old Age, With a Little Help," *New York Times*, December 12, 2012, accessed August 20, 2016, http://well.blogs.nytimes.com/2012/12/24/staying-independent-in-old-age-with-a-little-help/?_r=0.

6. Jules Rosen, MD, "A Doctor's View: Depression in Long Term Care Residents," *Health Progress*, Catholic Health Association of the United States, November–December 2014, accessed August 20, 2016, https://www.chausa.org/publications/health-progress/article/november-december-2014/a-doctor's-view-depression-in-long-term-care-res.

7. Rick Schmitt, "The Stranger in Your Home," *AARP Bulletin* 56, no. 2 (March 2015).

2. GETTING STARTED

1. Medicare, "Your Medicare Coverage. Home Health Services," accessed December 2, 2016, https://www.medicare.gov/coverage/home-health-services.html.

2. AARP, the Commonwealth Fund, and the Scan Foundation, "Raising Expectations 2014: The Scorecard on Long-Term Services and Supports for Older Adults, People with Physical Disabilities, and Family Caregivers," accessed January 19, 2017, http://www.longtermscorecard.org/.

3. Judith Graham, "Older People Become What They Think, Study Shows," *New York Times*, December 19, 2012, accessed December 2, 2016, http://newoldage.blogs.nytimes.com/2012/12/19/older-people-are-what-they-think-study-shows/?_r=0eve.

4. Becky Levy, "Ageism, Attitude, and Health. Buying into Old Age Putdown Is Bad for You: Here's Why," *US News and World Report*, December 26, 2015, accessed August 21, 2016, http://health.usnews.com/health-news/health-wellness/articles/2015-12-26/ageism-attitude-and-health.

5. Genworth, "Compare Long Term Care Costs Across the United States," accessed August 21, 2016, https://www.genworth.com/about-us/industry-expertise/cost-of-care.htmlenworth.

6. Tim Mullaney, "Where Home Care Rates Are Rising Most Sharply," *Home Health Care News*, accessed August 21, 2016, http://homehealthcare news.com/2016/05/where-home-care-rates-are-rising-most-sharply/.

7. California Department of Health Care Services, "Do You Qualify for Medi-Cal Benefits?" accessed August 21, 2016, http://www.dhcs.ca.gov/services/medi-cal/Pages/DoYouQualifyForMedi-Cal.aspx.

3. FINDING THE RIGHT HIRED CAREGIVER FOR YOU AND YOUR FAMILY

1. Paraprofessional Healthcare Institute, "Personal Care Aide Training Requirements," accessed August 22, 2016, http://phinational.org/policy/issues/training-credentialing/training-requirements-state/personal-care-aide-training.

2. New York State Division of Licensing Services, "FAQ's Cosmetology," accessed August 22, 2016, http://www.dos.ny.gov/licensing/cosmetology/cosmetology_faq.html.

3. Susan C. Reinhard et al., "Raising Expectations: AARP State Scorecard on Long Term Services and Supports for Older Adults, People with Disabilities, and Family Caregivers," June 2014.

4. Paraprofessional Healthcare Institute, "Training and Credentialing," accessed August 22, 2016, www.phinational.org/policy/issues/training-credentialing.

5. Bureau of Labor Statistics, "Occupational Outlook Handbook/Personal Care Aides," accessed August 22, 2016, http://www.bls.gov/ooh/personal-care-and-service/personal-care-aides.htm.

6. National Alliance for Caregiving, "Caregiving in the U.S. 2015," accessed August 22, 2016, http://www.caregiving.org/caregiving2015/.

7. Paraprofessional Healthcare Institute, "Growing Demand for Direct Care Workers," accessed August 22, 2016, http://phinational.org/growing-demand-direct-care-workers.

8. Judith Graham, "A Shortage of Caregivers," *New York Times*, February 26, 2014, accessed August 22, 2016, http://newoldage.blogs.nytimes.com/2014/02/26/a-shortage-of-caregivers/?_r=0.

9. Jennifer Ortman, Victoria A. Velkoff, and Howard Hogan, "An Aging Nation: The Older Population in the United States: Population Estimates and Projections Current Population Reports," U.S. Department of Commerce Economics and Statistics Administration, U.S. Census Bureau, May 2014, 25–1140.

10. Bureau of Labor Statistics, "Occupational Outlook Handbook/Personal Care Aides."

11. Alzheimer's Association, "Alzheimer's Association 2016 Alzheimer's Disease Facts and Figures," accessed August 22, 2016, http://www.alz.org/facts/.

12. N. A. Kramer and M. C. Smith, "Training Nursing Assistants to Care for Nursing Home Residents with Dementia," in *Professional Psychology in Long-Term Care* (New York: Hatherleigh Press, 2000), 227–56.

13. U.S. Equal Employment Opportunity Commission, "Background Checks: What Job Applicants and Employees Should Know," accessed August 21, 2016, https://www.eeoc.gov/eeoc/publications/background_checks_employees.cfm.

14. Fair Credit Reporting Act, 15 U.S.C§1681, September 2012, accessed August 21, 2016, https://www.consumer.ftc.gov/sites/default/files/articles/pdf/pdf-0111-fair-credit-reporting-act.pdf.

15. Care.com, "The Background on Background Checks," accessed August 29, 2016, https://www.care.com/background-checks.

16. Federal Bureau of Investigation, "Identity History Summary Checks," *Criminal Justice Information Services*, accessed August 20, 2016, https://www.fbi.gov/services/cjis/identity-history-summary-checks.

17. My FBI Report, Government Authorized, FBI Approved Channeler for FBI Records, accessed August 20, 2016, http://www.myfbireport.com/index.php.

4. BUILDING THE BEST CARE PARTNERSHIP

1. Alzheimer's Association, "What Is Dementia?" accessed September 8, 2016, http://www.alz.org/what-is-dementia.asp.

2. Private Duty Insider, "Private Duty Home Care State Licensing Laws," accessed September 8, 2016, http://privateduty.decisionhealth.com/State-Laws.aspx.

3. Franchise Business Review, "Top Senior Care Franchises," accessed September 8, 2016, www.franchisebusinessreview.com/franchise-reports/top-senior-care-franchises/.

4. Catalyst, "Top 10 Female-Dominated U.S. Occupations," accessed September 8, 2016, http://www.catalyst.org/knowledge/women-male-dominated-industries-and-occupations.

5. Mary Beth Sammons, "10 Caregiving Apps, Tech and Sites that Are Improving the Caregiving Experience," *CareNovate Magazine*, July 26, 2016, accessed August 30, 2016, http://carenovatemag.com/technology-and-caregiving/.

6. CareZone.com, Home Page, accessed August 30, 2016, https://carezone.com/home.

7. Jim Handy, "Does the 'Do Not Call' List Even Work?" *Forbes/Tech*, accessed August 29, 2016, http://www.forbes.com/sites/jimhandy/2013/02/27/does-the-do-not-call-list-even-work/#4230f2ac1175.

8. Geoff Williams, "How to Protect Your Elderly Parents from Being Scammed," *US News and World Report Money*, April 10, 2013, accessed August 27, 2016, http://money.usnews.com/money/personal-finance/articles/2013/04/10/how-to-protect-your-elderly-parents-from-being-scammed.

5. KEEP YOUR EYE ON THE BALL

1. Knapton Insurance, "How to Prepare a Home Inventory," May 23, 2013, accessed September 8, 2016, http://www.knaptoninsurance.com/how-to-prepare-a-home-inventory/.

2. Ray Martin, "12 Things to Keep at a Safe at Home, Not at a Bank," *CBS Moneywatch*, January 18, 2012, accessed September 8, 2016, http://www.cbsnews.com/news/12-things-to-keep-in-a-safe-at-home-not-at-a-bank/.

3. Dale Russakoff, "Guns in Frail Hands," *New York Times*, July 14, 2010, accessed September 9, 2016, http://newoldage.blogs.nytimes.com/2010/07/14/guns-in-frail-hands/?_r=0.

4. Brian Mertens and Susan B. Sorenson, "Current Considerations about the Elderly and Firearms," *American Journal of Public Health*, March 2012, accessed September 9, 2016, http://ajph.aphapublications.org/doi/abs/10.2105/AJPH.2011.300404.

5. Victoria Stunt, "Use of Surveillance Tech to Monitor Seniors at Home on Rise," *CBC News*, March 9, 2014, accessed September 10, 2016, http://www.cbc.ca/news/technology/use-of-surveillance-tech-to-monitor-seniors-at-home-on-rise-1.2535677.

6. Jim T. Miller, "How to Keep Tabs on an Elderly Parent with Video Monitoring," *Huffington Post*, January 11, 2016, accessed September 9, 2016, http://www.huffingtonpost.com/jim-t-miller/how-to-keep-tabs-on-an-el-el_b_8954044.html.

7. Chris Serres, "Hidden 'Granny Cams' Spread in Popularity as Weapon in Catching Elder Abuse," *Star Tribune*, March 14, 2016, accessed September 12, 2016, http://www.startribune.com/hidden-granny-cams-spread-in-popularity-as-weapon-for-catching-elder-abuse/371935611/.

8. WatchBot, "Elderly Care Camera," accessed September 2016, http://www.watchbotcamera.com/elderly-care/.

9. Youtube, "Caught on Camera: A Caretaker Abuses a 94 Year Old Woman," accessed September 15, 2016, https://www.youtube.com/watch?v=P2TcyHYWKwI.

10. Youtube, "Elder Abuse Caught on Tape, Mission Viejo, CA," accessed September 15, 2016, https://www.youtube.com/watch?v=Ta3tVKbT1DU.

11. DailyMail.com, "Shocking Video from Nursing Home Shows Abuse of Elderly Patient," accessed September 15, 2016, http://www.dailymail.co.uk/video/news/video-1008884/Shocking-video-nursing-home-shows-abuse-elderly-patient.html.

12. Rick Schmitt, "Elder Abuse: When Caregiving Goes Wrong," *AARP Bulletin*, March 2015, accessed September 12, 2016, http://www.aarp.org/home-family/caregiving/info-2015/elder-abuse-assisted-living.html.

13. National Center on Elder Abuse, "Red Flags of Neglect," accessed September 3, 2016, https://ncea.acl.gov/resources/docs/Red-Flags-Elder-Abuse-NCEA-2015.pdf.

14. National Neighborhood Watch, A Division of the National Sheriffs' Organization, "Medication Theft: Protecting Our Most Vulnerable Neighbors," accessed September 19, 2016, http://www.nnw.org/publication/medication-theft-protecting-our-most-vulnerable-neighbors.

15. Truelink, "The Truelink Report on Elder Financial Abuse 2015," accessed October 6, 2016, https://www.cambiahealth.com/sites/default/files/resources/whitepapers/The%20True%20Link%20Report%20on%20Elder%20Financial%20Abuse%202015_0.pdf.

16. National Adult Protective Services Association, "Elder Financial Exploitation," accessed October 6, 2016, http://www.napsa-now.org/policy-advocacy/exploitation/.

17. U.S. Department of Justice, "Elder Abuse FAQS: Warning Signs," accessed October 6, 2016, https://www.justice.gov/elderjustice/support/faq.

18. Geoff Williams, "How to Protect Your Elderly Parents from Being Scammed," *US News and World Report Money*, April 10, 2013, accessed August 27, 2016, http://money.usnews.com/money/personal-finance/articles/2013/04/10/how-to-protect-your-elderly-parents-from-being-scammed.

19. Ibid.

20. Merriam-Webster Dictionary, "Denial," accessed September 14, 2016, http://www.merriam-webster.com/dictionary/denial.

21. National Association of Adult Protective Services Administrators, "Survey Report: Problems Facing State Adult Protective Services Programs and the Resources Needed to Resolve Them," January 2003, accessed September 15, 2016, https://ncea.acl.gov/resources/docs/archive/Problems-Facing-Adults-APS-2003.pdf.

22. M. DeLiema et al., "Voices from the Frontlines: Examining Elder Abuse from Multiple Professional Perspectives," *Health and Social Work*, 40, no. 2 (April 2015): e15–e24.

23. The Philadelphia Corporation for Aging and the National Adult Protective Services Association, "2013 Federal Interagency guidance on Privacy Laws and Reporting Financial Abuse of Older Adults," accessed October 14, 2016, http://www.nyselderabuse.org/documents/Guidelines.pdf.

6. YOUR HOME, YOUR CARE

1. Crystal Galyean, "The Imperfect Rise of the American Suburbs," accessed December 2, 2016, http://ushistoryscene.com/article/levittown/.

2. Atul Gawande, *Being Mortal: Medicine and What Matters in the End* (New York: Metropolitan Books, Henry Holt and Company, 2014), 17.

3. Tribune News Service Contact Reporter, "We All Want to Die with Dignity—But Not Yet," *Chicago Tribune*, March 8, 2016, http://www.chicagotribune.com/lifestyles/health/ct-end-of-life-health-20160308-story.html.

4. Paula Span, "Complexities of Choosing an End Game for Dementia," *New York Times*, January 19, 2015, accessed October 17, 2016, http://www.nytimes.com/2015/01/20/health/complexities-of-choosing-an-end-game-for-dementia.html.

5. Ezekiel J. Emanuel, "Why I Hope to Die at 75," *The Atlantic*, October 2014, accessed October 17, 2016, http://www.theatlantic.com/magazine/archive/2014/10/why-i-hope-to-die-at-75/379329/.

6. Elspeth Slayter Recevik, "Twinkies for Breakfast: Implementing the Dignity of Risk with Adults with Intellectual Disabilities," *Disability Info*, accessed November 11, 2016, http://www.disabilityinfo.org.

7. Alice Page and Kim Marheine, "The Dignity of Risk: Balancing Rights, Self Determination and Risk in Supported Decision Making," presented at In Control Wisconsin: Aging Empowerment 2016, Madison, Wisconsin, June 8, 2016.

8. Ibid.

9. National Adult Protective Services Association, "2013 Nationwide Survey of Mandatory Reporting Requirements for Elderly and/or Vulnerable Persons," accessed November 11, 2016, http://www.napsa-now.org/wp-content/uploads/2014/11/Mandtory-Reporting-Chart-updated-Final.pdf.

10. National Adult Protective Services Association, "Code of Ethics," accessed November 11, 2016, http://www.napsa-now.org.

11. Full Circle America, accessed November 1, 2016, http://www.fullcircleamerica.com.

12. Allen S. Teel, *Alone and Invisible No More: How Grassroots Community Action and 21st Century Technologies Can Empower Elders to Stay in Their Homes and Lead Healthier, Happier Lives* (White River Junction, VT: Chelsea Green Publishing, 2011), 140.

13. American Psychological Association, "Assessment of Older Adults with Diminished Capacity. A Handbook for Psychologists," accessed November 11, 2016, http://www.apa.org/pi/agingprograms/assessment/capacity-psychologist-handbook.pdf.

14. Aanaand Naik et al., "Accessing Capacity in Suspected Cases of Self-Neglect," *Geriatrics*, accessed November 11, 2016, http://www.ncbi.nlm.nih.gov/pmc/articles/PMC2847362.

15. National Guardianship Association, "Questions and Answers on Guardianship Issues," accessed November 11, 2016, http://www.guardianship.org.

16. Health Care Providers Insurance Organization, "A Question of Refusing to Care for a Patient," accessed November 11, 2016, http://www.hpso.com/risk-education/individuals/articles.

7. THE CAREGIVER RELATIONSHIP

1. National Alliance for Caregiving, "Caregiving in the U.S. 2015," accessed November 4, 2016, http://www.aarp.org/content/dam/aarp/ppi/2015/caregiving-in-the-united-states-2015-report-revised.pdf.

2. Ibid.

3. Philip Moeller, "5 Steps to a Family Caregiver Agreement," *US News and World Report*, September 6, 2011, accessed November 10, 2016, http://money.usnews.com/money/blogs/the-best-life/2011/09/06/5-steps-to-a-family-caregiving-agreement.

4. *The Merriam-Webster Dictionary* (Springfield, MA: Merriam Webster Incorporated, 2004), 573.

5. World Privacy Forum, "Patient's Guide to HIPAA: Which Healthcare Entities Must Comply with HIPAA?" accessed April 10, 2017, https://www.worldprivacyforum.org/2013/09/hipaaguide9-2/.

6. Care.com Senior CareTeam, "Hiring Caregivers Guide: Senior Caregiver Interview Tips," accessed November 5, 2016, https://www.care.com/senior-care-senior-caregiver-interview-tips-p1145-q7744646.html; Rebecca Colmer, "Top 25 Interview Questions You Should Ask a Potential Caregiver," *Seniors Resource Guide*, accessed November 5, 2016, http://www.seniorsresourceguide.com/articles/art00980.html.

7. Nursing Home Care Standards, California Advocates for Nursing Home Reform, *Long Term Care Justice and Advocacy*, accessed November 6, 2016, http://www.canhr.org/factsheets/nh_fs/html/fs_CareStandards.html.

8. Julia Quinn-Szcesuil, "Sample Adult and Senior Care Contract," accessed November 11, 2016, https://www.care.com/c/stories/5429/sample-adult-and-senior-care-contract/.

8. THROWING IN THE TOWEL

1. Carolyn Said, "Honor Lands $20 Million for Senior In Home Care," *San Francisco Chronicle*, April 2, 2015.

2. Genworth, "Compare Long Term Care Costs Across the United States," accessed November 28, 2016, https://www.genworth.com/about-us/industry-expertise/cost-of-care.html.

3. American Health Care Association, "Assisted Living 2016 State Regulatory Review," accessed November 28, 2016, https://www.ahcancal.org/ncal/resources/pages/assistedlivingregulations.aspx.

4. Centers for Disease Control and Prevention, "National Survey of Residential Care Facilities," accessed November 28, 2016, http://www.cdc.gov/nchs/nsrcf/.

5. Paula Span, "Studies Find Mixed Results for Dementia Units," *New York Times*, May 10, 2013, accessed November 21, 2016, http://newoldage.blogs. nytimes.com/2013/05/10/dementia-care-units-may-improve-care-studies-suggest/?_r=0.

6. Johns Hopkins Medicine, "Living at Home with Dementia," *John Hopkins Medicine News and Publications*, December 17, 2013, accessed November 22, 2016, http://www.hopkinsmedicine.org/news/media/releases/living_at_home_with_dementia.

7. Alzheimer's Association, "Alzheimer's Association 2016 Alzheimer's Disease Facts and Figures," accessed November 22, 2016, http://www.alz.org/facts/, 5.

8. Michael Sandler, "New Living Arrangements for Dementia Patients," *Modern Healthcare*, March 19, 2016, accessed November 21, 2016, http://www.modernhealthcare.com/article/20160319/MAGAZINE/303199980.

9. Ibid.

10. Paying for Senior Care, "Senior Care Costs/Aging Care Calculator," accessed November 21, 2016, https://www.payingforseniorcare.com/longtermcare/costs.html#title5.

11. Georgia Burke and Gwen Orlowski, "Training to Serve People with Dementia: Is Our Health Care System Ready?" *Justice in Aging*, Issue Brief, August 2015, accessed November 21, 2016, http://www.justiceinaging.org/wp-content/uploads/2015/08/Training-to-serve-people-with-dementia-Alz2FINAL.pdf.

12. A. Kelly et al., "Length of Stay for Older Adults in Nursing Homes at the End of Life," *Journal of American Geriatric Society* 58, no. 9 (September 2010): 1701–6.

9. CREATIVE SOLUTIONS

1. Washington State Department of Social and Health Services, "About Adult Family Homes," accessed December 3, 2016, https://www.dshs.wa.gov/altsa/residential-care-services/about-adult-family-homes.

2. California Registry, "Residential Care Homes (AKA Board and Care)," accessed December 3, 2016, http://www.calregistry.com/housing/bce.htm.

3. Tina Rosenberg, "Reviving House Calls by Doctors," *New York Times*, September 27, 2016, accessed December 10, 2016, http://www.nytimes.com/2016/09/27/opinion/reviving-house-calls-by-doctors.html?_r=0.

4. Ibid.

5. Matt Zavadsky et al., "Mobile Integrated Healthcare and Community Paramedicine," National Association of Emergency Medical Technicians, accessed December 10, 2016, http://www.naemt.org/docs/default-source/community-paramedicine/naemt-mih-cp-report.pdf?sfvrsn=4.

6. Ibid.

7. Beth Baker, *With a Little Help from Our Friends: Creating Community as We Grow Older* (Nashville: Vanderbilt University Press, 2014).

8. Marilyn Bowden, "A Plan for Aging in Place," Bankrate.com, accessed December 10, 2016, http://www.bankrate.com/finance/retirement/naturally-occurring-retirement-communities-1.aspx.

9. Paying for Senior Care, "Medicare PACE/LIFE Program Provider List—2016," accessed December 3, 2016, https://www.payingforseniorcare.com/long-termcare/resources/pace_medicare/provider_list.html.

10. Medicare, "PACE," Medicare.gov, accessed December 3, 2016, https://www.medicare.gov/your-medicare-costs/help-paying-costs/pace/pace.html.

11. National PACE Association, "Research," accessed December 3, 2016, http://www.npaonline.org/policy-advocacy/state-policy/research.

12. M. D. Fretwell et al., "The Elderhaus Program of All-Inclusive Care for the Elderly in North Carolina: Improving Functional Outcomes and Reducing Cost of Care: Preliminary Data," *Journal of American Geriatric Society* 3, no. 3 (March 2015): 578–83; National PACE Association, "Research."

13. Sarah Varney, "Private Equity Pursues Profits in Keeping the Elderly at Home," *New York Times*, August 20, 2016, accessed January 5, 2017, http://www.nytimes.com/2016/08/21/business/as-the-for-profit-world-moves-into-an-elder-care-program-some-worry.html.

14. Ibid.

15. National Shared Housing Resource Center, "About National Shared Housing Resource," accessed December 9, 2016, http://nationalsharedhousing.org/news/.

16. MetLife Mature Market Institute, "The MetLife National Study of Adult Day Services: Providing Support to Individuals and Their Family Caregivers," October 2010, accessed January 5, 2017, https://www.metlife.com/assets/cao/mmi/publications/studies/2010/mmi-adult-day-services.pdf.

17. Ibid.

18. Ibid.

19. U-Exchange, "Legalities of Bartering," accessed January 5, 2017, http://www.u-exchange.com/bartering-legalities.

20. Jenni Bergal, "Tax Credits for Ramps, Grab Bars to Help Seniors Stay at Home," *Stateline: The Pew Charitable Trusts*, August 24, 2016, accessed December 14, 2016, http://www.pewtrusts.org/en/research-and-analysis/blogs/

stateline/2016/08/24/tax-credits-for-ramps-grab-bars-to-help-seniors-stay-at-home.

21. Jennifer Ludden, "Building Homes to Age In," *National Public Radio*, August 24, 2010, accessed January 5, 2017, http://www.npr.org/templates/story/story.php?storyId=129260583.

22. Bergal, "Tax Credits for Ramps, Grab Bars to Help Seniors Stay at Home."

23. Paraprofessional Healthcare Institute, "What Are the Challenges for This Workforce?" accessed December 10, 2016, http://phinational.org/sites/phinational.org/files/phi-home-care-workers-key-facts.pdf.

24. Honor.com, "Caring for Our Care Pros: Honor Announces a Huge Change," January 19, 2016, accessed December 8, 2016, https://blog.joinhonor.com/2016/01/19/caring-for-care-pros/.

25. Ai-Jen Poo, with Ariane Conrad, *The Age of Dignity: Preparing for the Elder Boom in a Changing America* (New York: New Press, 2015), 146–47.

BIBLIOGRAPHY

AARP Public Policy Institute. "Aging in Place. A State Survey of Livability Policies and Practices." A Research Report by the National Conference of State Legislatures and the AARP Public Policy Institute. Accessed December 2, 2016. http://assets.aarp.org/rgcenter/ppi/liv-com/ib190.pdf.

AARP, the Commonwealth Fund, and the Scan Foundation. "Raising Expectations 2014: The Scorecard on Long-Term Services and Supports for Older Adults, People with Physical Disabilities, and Family Caregivers." Accessed January 19, 2017. http://www.longtermscorecard.org/.

Alzheimer's Association. "Alzheimer's Association 2016 Alzheimer's Disease Facts and Figures." Accessed August 22, 2016. http://www.alz.org/facts/.

———. "What Is Dementia?" Accessed September 8, 2016. http://www.alz.org/what-is-dementia.asp.

American Elder Care Research Organization. "Senior Care Costs/Aging Care Calculator. Paying for Senior Care: Understand Your Options for Long Term Care." Accessed November 21, 2016. https://www.payingforseniorcare.com/longtermcare/costs.html#title5.

American Health Care Association. "Assisted Living 2016 State Regulatory Review." Accessed November 28, 2016. https://www.ahcancal.org/ncal/resources/pages/assistedlivingregulations.aspx.

American Psychological Association. "Assessment of Older Adults with Diminished Capacity. A Handbook for Psychologists." Accessed November 11, 2016. http://www.apa.org/pi/agingprograms/assessment/capacity-psychologist-handbook.pdf.

Baker, Beth. *With a Little Help from Our Friends: Creating Community as We Grow Older.* Nashville: Vanderbilt University Press, 2014.

Bergal, Jenni. "Tax Credits for Ramps, Grab Bars to Help Seniors Stay at Home." *Stateline: The Pew Charitable Trusts.* August 24, 2016. Accessed December 14, 2016. http://www.pewtrusts.org/en/research-and-analysis/blogs/stateline/2016/08/24/tax-credits-for-ramps-grab-bars-to-help-seniors-stay-at-home.

Bowden, Marilyn. "A Plan for Aging in Place." Bankrate.com. Accessed December 10, 2016. http://www.bankrate.com/finance/retirement/naturally-occurring-retirement-communities-1.aspx.

Brody, Jane. "Staying Independent in Old Age, With a Little Help." *New York Times.* December 12, 2012. Accessed August 20, 2016. http://well.blogs.nytimes.com/2012/12/24/staying-independent-in-old-age-with-a-little-help/.

Bureau of Labor Statistics. "Occupational Outlook Handbook/Personal Care Aides." Accessed August 22, 2016. http://www.bls.gov/ooh/personal-care-and-service/personal-care-aides.htm.

Burke, Georgia, and Gwen Orlowski. "Training to Serve People with Dementia: Is Our Health Care System Ready?" *Justice in Aging.* Issue Brief. August 2015. Accessed November 21, 2016. http://www.justiceinaging.org/wp-content/uploads/2015/08/Training-to-serve-people-with-dementia-Alz2FINAL.pdf.

California Department of Health Care Services. "Do you Qualify for Medi-Cal Benefits?" Accessed August 21, 2016. http://www.dhcs.ca.gov/services/mhttp://homehealthcare-news.com/2016/05/where-home-care-rates-are-rising-most-sharply/edi-cal/Pages/DoYou-QualifyForMedi-Cal.aspx.

California Nursing Home Abuse Lawyer Blog. "States Move toward Implementing Surveillance in Nursing Homes." Law Offices of Ben Yeroushamlmi, APC. December 16, 2013. Accessed September 10, 2016. http://www.californianursinghomeabuselawyer-blog.com/2013/12/states-move-toward-implementing-surveillance-in-nursing-homes.html.

California Registry. "Residential Care Homes (AKA Board and Care)." Accessed December 3, 2016. http://www.calregistry.com/housing/bce.htm.

Care.com. "The Background on Background Checks." Accessed August 29, 2016. https://www.care.com/background-checks.

Care.com Senior Care Team. "Hiring Caregivers Guide: Senior Caregiver Interview Tips." Accessed November 5, 2016. https://www.care.com/senior-care-senior-caregiver-interview-tips-p1145-q7744646.html.

CareZone.com. Home Page. Accessed August 30, 2016. https://carezone.com/home.

Catalyst. "Top 10 Female-Dominated U.S. Occupations." Accessed September 8, 2016. http://www.catalyst.org/knowledge/women-male-dominated-industries-and-occupations.

Centers for Disease Control and Prevention. "National Survey of Residential Care Facilities." Accessed November 28, 2016. http://www.cdc.gov/nchs/nsrcf/.

Colmer, Rebecca. "Top 25 Interview Questions You Should Ask a Potential Caregiver." *Seniors Resource Guide.* Accessed November 5, 2016. http://www.seniorsresourceguide.com/articles/art00980.html.

DailyMail.com. "Shocking Video from Nursing Home Shows Abuse of Elderly Patient." Accessed September 15, 2016. http://www.dailymail.co.uk/video/news/video-1008884/Shocking-video-nursing-home-shows-abuse-elderly-patient.html.

Decision Health. "Private Duty Home Care State Licensing Laws." Accessed September 8, 2016. http://privateduty.decisionhealth.com/StateLaws.aspx.

DeLiema, M., A. Navarro, S. Enguidanos, and K. Wilber. "Voices from the Frontlines: Examining Elder Abuse from Multiple Professional Perspectives." *Health and Social Work* 40, no. 2 (April 2015): e15–e24. Accessed September 15, 2016. https://www.researchgate.net/publication/273912416_Voices_from_the_Frontlines_Examining_Elder_Abuse_from_Multiple_Professional_Perspectives.

Emanuel, Ezekiel J. "Why I Hope to Die at 75." *The Atlantic.* October 2014. Accessed October 17, 2016. http://www.theatlantic.com/magazine/archive/2014/10/why-i-hope-to-die-at-75/379329/.

Emergency Medical Technicians. Accessed December 10, 2016. http://www.naemt.org/docs/default-source/community-paramedicine/naemt-mih-cp-report.pdf?sfvrsn=4.

Fair Credit Reporting Act. 15 U.S.C§1681. September 2012. Accessed August 21, 2016. https://www.consumer.ftc.gov/sites/default/files/articles/pdf/pdf-0111-fair-credit-reporting-act.pdf.

Federal Bureau of Investigation. "Identity History Summary Checks." *Criminal Justice Information Services.* Accessed August 20, 2016. https://www.fbi.gov/services/cjis/identity-history-summary-checks.

Franchise Business Review. "Top Senior Care Franchises." Accessed September 8, 2016. www.franchisebusinessreview.com/franchise-reports/top-senior-care-franchises/.

Fretwell, M. D., J. S. Old, K. Zwan, and K. Simhadre. "The Elderhaus Program of All-Inclusive Care for the Elderly in North Carolina: Improving Functional Outcomes and Reducing Cost of Care: Preliminary Data." *Journal of American Geriatric Society* 3, no. 3 (March 2015): 578–83.

Full Circle America. Accessed November 1, 2016. http://www.fullcircleamerica.com/.

Galyean, Crystal. "The Imperfect Rise of the American Suburbs." Accessed December 2, 2016. http://ushistoryscene.com/article/levittown/.

Genworth. "Compare Long Term Care Costs Across the United States." Accessed November 28, 2016. https://www.genworth.com/about-us/industry-expertise/cost-of-care.html.

Graham, Judith. "A Shortage of Caregivers." *New York Times.* February 26, 2014. Accessed August 22, 2016. http://newoldage.blogs.nytimes.com/2014/02/26/a-shortage-of-caregivers/?_r=0.

———. "Older People Become What They Think, Study Shows." *New York Times.* December 19, 2012. Accessed December 2, 2016. http://newoldage.blogs.nytimes.com/2012/12/19/older-people-are-what-they-think-study-shows/?_r=0eve What They Think, Study Shows.

Gawande, Atul. *Being Mortal: Medicine and What Matters in the End.* New York: Metropolitan Books, Henry Holt and Company, 2014.

Handy, Jim. "Does the 'Do Not Call' List Even Work?" *Forbes/Tech.* Accessed August 29, 2016. http://www.forbes.com/sites/jimhandy/2013/02/27/does-the-do-not-call-list-even-work/#4230f2ac1175.

Health Care Providers Insurance Organization. "A Question of Refusing to Care for a Patient." Accessed November 11, 2016. http://www.hpso.com/risk-education/individuals/articles.

Johns Hopkins Medicine. "Living at Home with Dementia." *Johns Hopkins Medicine News and Publications.* December 17, 2013. Accessed November 22, 2016. http://www.hopkinsmedicine.org/news/media/releases/living_at_home_with_dementia.

Kelly, A., J. Conell-Price, K. Covinsky, I. S. Cenzer, A. Chang, W. J. Boscardin, and A. K. Smith. "Length of Stay for Older Adults in Nursing Homes at the End of Life." *Journal of American Geriatric Society* 58, no. 9 (September 2010): 1701–6.

Knapton Insurance. "How to Prepare a Home Inventory." knaptoninsurance.com. May 23, 2013. Accessed September 8, 2016. http://www.knaptoninsurance.com/how-to-prepare-a-home-inventory/.

Kramer, N. A., and M. C. Smith. "Training Nursing Assistants to Care for Nursing Home Residents with Dementia." In *Professional Psychology in Long-Term Care,* edited by V. Molinari, 227–56. New York: Hatherleigh Press, 2000.

Levy, Becky. "Ageism, Attitude, and Health. Buying into Old Age Putdown Is Bad for You: Here's Why." *US News and World Report.* December 26, 2015. Accessed August 21, 2016. http://health.usnews.com/health-news/health-wellness/articles/2015-12-26/ageism-attitude-and-health.

Ludden, Jennifer. "Building Homes to Age In." *National Public Radio.* August 24, 2010. Accessed January 5, 2017. http://www.npr.org/templates/story/story.php?storyId=129260583.

Martin, Ray. "12 Things to Keep at a Safe at Home, Not at a Bank." *CBS Moneywatch.* January 18, 2012. Accessed September 8, 2016. http://www.cbsnews.com/news/12-things-to-keep-in-a-safe-at-home-not-at-a-bank/.

Medicare. "PACE." Accessed December 3, 2016. https://www.medicare.gov/your-medicare-costs/help-paying-costs/pace/pace.html.

———. "Your Medicare Coverage. Home Health Services." Accessed December 2, 2016. https://www.medicare.gov/coverage/home-health-services.htmles.

Merriam-Webster Dictionary. "Denial." Accessed September 14, 2016. http://www.merriam-webster.com/dictionary/denial, 573.

Mertens, Brian, and Susan B. Sorenson. "Current Considerations about the Elderly and Firearms." *American Journal of Public Health.* March 2012. Accessed September 9, 2016. http://ajph.aphapublications.org/doi/abs/10.2105/AJPH.2011.300404.

MetLife Mature Market Institute. "The MetLife National Study of Adult Day Services: Providing Support to Individuals and Their Family Caregivers." October 2010. Accessed January 5, 2017. https://www.metlife.com/assets/cao/mmi/publications/studies/2010/mmi-adult-day-services.pdf.

Miller, Jim T. "How to Keep Tabs on an Elderly Parent with Video Monitoring." *Huffington Post.* January 11, 2016. Accessed September 9, 2016. http://www.huffingtonpost.com/jim-t-miller/how-to-keep-tabs-on-an-el_b_8954044.html.

Moeller, Philip. "5 Steps to a Family Caregiver Agreement." *US News and World Report.* September 6, 2011. Accessed November 10, 2016. http://money.usnews.com/money/blogs/the-best-life/2011/09/06/5-steps-to-a-family-caregiving-agreement.

Mullaney, Tim. "Where Home Care Rates Are Rising Most Sharply." *Home Health Care News.* Accessed August 21, 2016. http://homehealthcarenews.com/2016/05/where-home-care-rates-are-rising-most-sharply/.

My FBI Report. "Government Authorized, FBI Approved Channeler for FBI Records." Accessed August 20, 2016. http://www.myfbireport.com/index.php.

Naik, Aanand, James M. Lai, Mark E. Kunik, and Carmel B. Dyer. "Accessing Capacity in Suspected Cases of Self-Neglect." *Geriatrics.* Accessed November 11, 2016. http://www.ncbi.nlm.nih.gov/pmc/articles/PMC2847362.

National Adult Protective Services Association. "Code of Ethics." Accessed November 11, 2016. http://www.napsa-now.org.

———. "Elder Financial Exploitation." Accessed October 6, 2016. http://www.napsa-now.org/policy-advocacy/exploitation/.

———. "2013 Nationwide Survey of Mandatory Reporting Requirements for Elderly and/or Vulnerable Persons." Accessed November 11, 2016. http://www.napsa-now.org/wp-content/uploads/2014/11/Mandtory-Reporting-Chart-updated-Final.pdf.

National Alliance for Caregiving. "Caregiving in the U.S. 2015." Accessed November 4, 2016. http://www.aarp.org/content/dam/aarp/ppi/2015/caregiving-in-the-united-states-2015-report-revised.pdf.

National Association of Adult Protective Services Administrators. "Survey Report: Problems Facing State Adult Protective Services Programs and the Resources Needed to Resolve Them." January 2003. Accessed September 15, 2016. https://ncea.acl.gov/resources/docs/archive/Problems-Facing-Adults-APS-2003.pdf.

National Center on Elder Abuse. "Red Flags of Neglect." Accessed September 3, 2016. https://ncea.acl.gov/resources/docs/Red-Flags-Elder-Abuse-NCEA-2015.pdf.

National Conference of State Legislatures and the AARP Public Policy Institute. "Aging in Place. A State Survey of Livability Policies and Practices." A Research Report by the National Conference of State Legislatures and the AARP Public Policy Institute. Accessed December 2, 2016. http://assets.aarp.org/rgcenter/ppi/liv-com/ib190.pdf.

National Guardianship Association. "Questions and Answers on Guardianship Issues." Accessed November 11, 2016. http://www.guardianship.org.

National Neighborhood Watch, A Division of the National Sheriffs' Organization. "Medication Theft: Protecting our Most Vulnerable Neighbors." Accessed September 19, 2016. http://www.nnw.org/publication/medication-theft-protecting-our-most-vulnerable-neighbors.

National PACE Association. "Research." Accessed December 3, 2016. http://www.npaonline.org/policy-advocacy/state-policy/research.

National Shared Housing Resource Center. "About National Shared Housing Resource." Accessed December 9, 2016. http://nationalsharedhousing.org/news/.

NBC Universal. "Home Health Aide Caught on Camera Abusing 78-Year-Old Stroke Victim." *NBC4 New York.* August 21, 2014. Accessed September 10, 2016. http://www.nbcnewyork.com/news/local/Health-Care-Aide-Abuse-Surveillance-Video-Stroke-Victim-Arrest-Personal-Touch-Queens-272005831.html.

New York State Coalition on Elder Abuse. "2013 Federal Interagency Guidance on Privacy Laws and Reporting Financial Abuse of Older Adults." Accessed October 14, 2016. http://www.nyselderabuse.org/documents/Guidelines.pdf.

New York State Division of Licensing Services. "FAQ's Cosmetology." Accessed August 22, 2016. http://www.dos.ny.gov/licensing/cosmetology/cosmetology_faq.html.

Nursing Home Care Standards. California Advocates for Nursing Home Reform. *Long Term Care Justice and Advocacy.* Accessed November 6, 2016. http://www.canhr.org/factsheets/nh_fs/html/fs_CareStandards.html.

Ortman, Jennifer, Victoria A. Velkoff, and Howard Hogan. "An Aging Nation: The Older Population in the United States: Population Estimates and Projections Current Population Reports." U.S. Department of Commerce Economics and Statistics Administration, U.S. Census Bureau, May 2014, 25–1140.

Page, Alice, and Kim Marheine. "The Dignity of Risk: Balancing Rights, Self Determination and Risk in Supported Decision Making." Paper presented at In Control Wisconsin: Aging Empowerment, Madison, Wisconsin, June 8, 2016.

Paraprofessional Healthcare Institute. "Growing Demand for Direct Care Workers." Accessed August 22, 2016. http://phinational.org/growing-demand-direct-care-workers.

———. "Personal Care Aide Training Requirements." Accessed August 22, 2016. http://phinational.org/policy/issues/training-credentialing/training-requirements-state/personal-care-aide-training.

———. "Report on How Poverty Wages Undermine Care." Accessed December 2, 2016. https://phinational.org/research-reports/paying-price-how-poverty-wages-undermine-home-care-america.

———. "Training and Credentialing." Accessed August 22, 2016. www.phinational.org/policy/issues/training-credentialing.

Paying for Senior Care. "Medicare PACE/LIFE Program Provider List—2016." Accessed December 3, 2016. https://www.payingforseniorcare.com/longtermcare/resources/pace_medicare/provider_list.html.

———. "Senior Care Costs/Aging Care Calculator." Accessed November 21, 2016. https://www.payingforseniorcare.com/longtermcare/costs.html#title5.

Poo, Ai-Jen, with Ariane Conrad. *The Age of Dignity: Preparing for the Elder Boom in a Changing America.* New York: New Press, 2015.

Private Duty Insider. "Private Duty Home Care State Licensing Laws." Accessed September 8, 2016. http://privateduty.decisionhealth.com/StateLaws.aspx.

Recevik, Elspeth Slayter. "Twinkies for Breakfast: Implementing the Dignity of Risk with Adults with Intellectual Disabilities." Disability Info. Accessed November 11, 2016. http://www.disabilityinfo.org.

Reinhard, Susan C., Enid Kassner, Ari Houser, Kathleen Ujvari, Robert Mollica, and Leslie Hendrickson. "Raising Expectations: AARP State Scorecard on Long Term Services and Supports for Older Adults, People with Disabilities, and Family Caregivers." June 2014.

Rosen, Jules, MD. "A Doctor's View: Depression in Long Term Care Residents." *Health Progress.* Catholic Health Association of the United States. November–December 2014. Accessed August 20, 2016. https://www.chausa.org/publications/health-progress/article/november-december-2014/a-doctor's-view-depression-in-long-term-care-res.

Rosenberg, Tina. "Reviving House Calls by Doctors." *New York Times.* September 27, 2016. Accessed December 10, 2016. http://www.nytimes.com/2016/09/27/opinion/reviving-house-calls-by-doctors.html?_r=0.

Russakoff, Dale. "Guns in Frail Hands." *New York Times.* July 14, 2010. Accessed September 9, 2016. http://newoldage.blogs.nytimes.com/2010/07/14/guns-in-frail-hands/?_r=0.

Said, Carolyn. "Honor Lands $20 Million for Senior in Home Care." *San Francisco Chronicle,* April 2, 2015.

Sammons, Mary Beth. "10 Caregiving Apps, Tech and Sites that Are Improving the Caregiving Experience." *CareNovate Magazine.* July 26, 2016. Accessed August 30, 2016. http://carenovatemag.com/technology-and-caregiving/.

Sandler, Michael. "New Living Arrangements for Dementia Patients." *Modern Healthcare.* March 19, 2016. Accessed November 21, 2016. http://www.modernhealthcare.com/article/20160319/MAGAZINE/303199980.

Schmitt, Rick. "Elder Abuse: When Caregiving Goes Wrong." *AARP Bulletin.* March 2015. Accessed September 12, 2016. http://www.aarp.org/home-family/caregiving/info-2015/elder-abuse-assisted-living.html.

———. "The Stranger in Your Home." *AARP Bulletin* 56, no. 2 (March 2015): 7–8.

Serres, Chris. "Hidden 'Granny Cams' Spread in Popularity as Weapon in Catching Elder Abuse." *Star Tribune.* March 14, 2016. Accessed September 12, 2016. http://www.startribune.com/hidden-granny-cams-spread-in-popularity-as-weapon-for-catching-elder-abuse/371935611/.

Span, Paula. "Complexities of Choosing an End Game for Dementia." *New York Times.* January 19, 2015. Accessed October 17, 2016. http://www.nytimes.com/2015/01/20/health/complexities-of-choosing-an-end-game-for-dementia.html.

———. "Studies Find Mixed Results for Dementia Units." *New York Times.* May 10, 2013. Accessed November 21, 2016. http://newoldage.blogs.nytimes.com/2013/05/10/dementia-care-units-may-improve-care-studies-suggest/?_r=0.

Stunt, Victoria. "Use of Surveillance Tech to Monitor Seniors at Home on Rise." *CBC News.* March 9, 2014. Accessed September 10, 2016. http://www.cbc.ca/news/technology/use-of-surveillance-tech-to-monitor-seniors-at-home-on-rise-1.2535677.

Teel, Allen S. *Alone and Invisible No More: How Grassroots Community Action and 21st Century Technologies Can Empower Elders to Stay in Their Homes and Lead Healthier, Happier Lives.* White River Junction City, VT: Chelsea Green Publishing, 2011.

The Philadelphia Corporation for Aging and the National Adult Protective Services Association. "2013 Federal Interagency Guidance on Privacy Laws and Reporting Financial Abuse of Older Adults." Accessed October 14, 2016. http://www.nyselderabuse.org/documents/Guidelines.pdf.

Tribune News Service Contact Reporter. "We All Want to Die with Dignity—But Not Yet." *Chicago Tribune.* March 8, 2016. http://www.chicagotribune.com/lifestyles/health/ct-end-of-life-health-20160308-story.html.

Truelink. "The Truelink Report on Elder Financial Abuse 2015." Accessed October 6, 2016. https://www.cambiahealth.com/sites/default/files/resources/whitepapers/The%20True%20Link%20Report%20on%20Elder%20Financial%20Abuse%202015_0.pdf.

Quinn-Szcesuil, Julia. "Sample Adult and Senior Care Contract." Accessed November 11, 2016. https://www.care.com/c/stories/5429/sample-adult-and-senior-care-contract/.

U-Exchange. "Legalities of Bartering." Accessed January 5, 2017. http://www.u-exchange.com/bartering-legalities.

U.S. Census Bureau. "Census Shows 65 and Older Population Growing Faster than Total U.S. Population." Accessed December 2, 2016. https://www.census.gov/newsroom/releases/archives/2010_census/cb11-cn192.html.

U.S. Department of Justice. "Elder Abuse FAQS: Warning Signs." Accessed October 6, 2016. https://www.justice.gov/elderjustice/support/faq.

U.S. Department of Veterans Affairs. "Medical Foster Home Care and Elder Veterans." Accessed December 3, 2016. http://www.va.gov/GERIATRICS/Guide/LongTermCare/Medical_Foster_Homes.asp.

U.S. Equal Employment Opportunity Commission. "Background Checks: What Job Applicants and Employees Should Know." Accessed August 21, 2016. https://www.eeoc.gov/eeoc/publications/background_checks_employees.cfm.

Varney, Sarah. "Private Equity Pursues Profits in Keeping the Elderly at Home." *New York Times.* August 20, 2016. Accessed January 5, 2017. http://www.nytimes.com/2016/08/21/business/as-the-for-profit-world-moves-into-an-elder-care-program-some-worry.html.

Washington State Department of Social and Health Services. "About Adult Family Homes." Accessed December 3, 2016. https://www.dshs.wa.gov/altsa/residential-care-services/about-adult-family-homes.

WatchBot. "Elderly Care Camera." Accessed September 2016. http://www.watchbotcamera.com/elderlcare/.

Williams, Geoff. "How to Protect Your Elderly Parents from Being Scammed." *US News and World Report Money.* April 10, 2013. Accessed August 27, 2016. http://money.usnews.com/money/personal-finance/articles/2013/04/10/how-to-protect-your-elderly-parents-from-being-scammed.

World Privacy Forum. "Patient's Guide to HIPAA: Which Healthcare Entities Must Comply with HIPAA?" Accessed April 10, 2017. https://www.worldprivacyforum.org/2013/09/hipaaguide9-2/.

Youtube. "Caught on Camera: A Caretaker Abuses a 94 Year Old Woman." Accessed September 15, 2016. https://www.youtube.com/watch?v=P2TcyHYWKwIcensus.gov.

———. "Elder Abuse Caught on Tape, Mission Viejo, CA." Accessed September 15, 2016. https://www.youtube.com/watch?v=Ta3tVKbT1DU.

Zavadsky, Matt, Troy Hagen, Paul Hinchey, Kevin McGinnis, Scott Bourn, and Brent Myers. "Mobile Integrated Healthcare and Community Paramedicine." National Association of

Emergency Medical Technicians. Accessed December 10, 2016. http://www.naemt.org/docs/default-source/community-paramedicine/naemt-mih-cp-report.pdf?sfvrsn=4.

INDEX